Life with the Pneumococcus

Life with the Pneumococcus

Notes from the Bedside, Laboratory, and Library

Robert Austrian, M.D.

Foreword by Lewis Thomas, M.D.

University of Pennsylvania Press
Philadelphia
1985

Library of Congress Cataloging in Publication Data

Austrian, Robert.
  Life with the pneumococcus.

  Articles reprinted from various journals.
  Includes bibliographies.
    1. Pneumococcal vaccine—Addresses, essays,
lectures. 2. Pneumonia, Pneumococcal—Prevention—
Addresses, essays, lectures. 3. Streptococcal
infections—Prevention—Addresses, essays, lectures.
4. Streptococcus pneumoniae—Addresses, essays,
lectures. I. Title. [DNLM: 1. Bacterial Vaccines—
immunology—collected works. 2. Bacterial Vaccines—
therapeutic use—collected works. 3. Pneumococcal
Infections—prevention & control—collected works.
4. Streptococcus Pneumoniae—immunology—collected
works. 5. Streptococcus Pneumoniae—pathogenicity—
collected works. WC 217 A938L]
QR189.5.P58A93 1985   616.9′2   85-1001
ISBN 0-8122-7977-8

Printed in the United States of America

Credits

Chapter 1: "Concerning Friedländer, Gram and the Etiology of Pneumonia, an Historical Note." *Transactions of the American Climatological Association*, vol. 71, pp. 142–149, 1959. Reprinted by permission of the American Clinical and Climatological Association.
(This paper was presented at the 72nd Annual Meeting of the American Clinical and Climatological Association, November 3, 1959.)
Chapter 2: "The Pneumococcus at Hopkins: Early Portents of Future Developments." *The Johns Hopkins Medical Journal*, vol. 144, pp. 192–201, 1979. Reprinted with permission.
(This paper was presented as the Thayer Lecture in Clinical Medicine, The Johns Hopkins University School of Medicine, March 15, 1979.)
Chapter 3: "The Quellung Reaction: A Neglected Microbiologic Technique." *The Mount Sinai Medical Journal*, vol. 43, No. 6, pp. 699–709, 1976. Reprinted with permission.
Chapter 4: "Random Gleanings from a Life with the Pneumococcus." *Journal of Infectious Diseases*, vol. 131, No. 4, pp. 474–484, 1975. © 1975 by the University of Chicago Press. All rights reserved. Reprinted by permission of the University of Chicago Press.
(This paper was presented at the annual meeting of the Infectious Diseases Society of America, September 10, 1974, San Francisco, CA. A Lecture in honor of Maxwell Finland.)
Chapter 5: "Pneumococcus: The First One Hundred Years." *Review of Infectious Diseases*, vol. 3, No.2, pp. 183–189, 1981. © 1981 by the University of Chicago Press. All rights reserved. Reprinted by permission of the University of Chicago Press.
Chapter 6: "The Current Status of Bacteremic Pneumococcal Pneumonia: Reevaluation of an Underemphasized Clinical Problem." Reprinted by permission of the *Transactions of the Association of American Physicians*, vol. LXXVI, pp. 117–124, 1963.
Chapter 7: "Prevention of Pneumococcal Pneumonia by Vaccination." Vol. 89, pp. 184–192, 1976. Reprinted by permission of the *Transactions of the Association of American Physicians*, vol. LXXXIX, pp. 184–192, 1976.
Chapter 8: "Of Gold and Pneumococci: A History of Pneumococcal Vaccines in South Africa." *Transactions of the American Clinical and Climatological Association*, vol. 89, pp. 141–161, 1977. Reprinted with permission of the American Clinical and Climatological Association.
(A Jeremiah Metzger Lecture)

To the memory of
CHARLES R. AUSTRIAN,
COLIN M. MACLEOD, and
W. BARRY WOOD, JR.,
without whose insights
and instruction these
vignettes would not have
been written.

Contents

Foreword

LEWIS THOMAS, M.D.

The major figures in American biomedical research come in several quite different classes. There are those who shift swiftly from problem to problem, sometimes leaping freely from one biological discipline to another and then back again, lighting finally on a soluble problem as though by accident. There are others who meditate on a single puzzle for years at a time, scarcely moving, and then, obsessed overnight by the idea of a lifetime, swoop down like nightowls on the single answer.

And there are those who pick out the one problem that will preoccupy them for an entire career of hard work and then just keep at it, year after year. This may seem the safest way to live a life in science, but it is actually, in real life, the chanciest of all gambles, like putting all your chips on a single number, play after play, until all your money runs out.

Robert Austrian's career has been this last kind. He became fascinated by a single microorganism, *Streptococcus pneumoniae*, long ago, and simply stuck with it. As the years went by, some of his colleagues came to believe that he was simply stuck with it. Finally, not as a result of good luck or any nocturnal revelation or unforeseen laboratory accident, but as the uncommon reward for steady, meticulous, logical experimentation, he got what he was after: a polyvalent vaccine against pneumococcal infection.

The papers in this book are a nice historical record of how science goes when it is going slowly but going well. They are also a lesson in what most savvy investigators take on faith: that if you can learn enough new things about living things at a fundamental level, sooner or later you may have the chance, as Austrian has had, to turn basic science into applied science and, at last, into a useful product.

Life with the Pneumococcus

"... et j'ai connu un homme qui prouvait, par de bonnes raisons, qu'il ne faut jamais dire: 'une telle personne est morte d'une fièvre et d'une fluxion sur la poitrine'; 'Elle est morte de quatre médicins et de deux apothicaires.'"

Molière, *L'Amour de Medicin*
Acte II, Scène II

1

The Gram Stain and the Etiology of Lobar Pneumonia: An Historical Note

Although the historical facts concerning the etiology of lobar pneumonia and Gram's original work on the widely used stain which now bears his name are well documented, an examination of the original reports of these two topics has brought to light an unusual facet of the story pertaining to them. It is a tale which re-emphasizes the widely quoted aphorism of Pasteur that chance favors only the prepared mind. The polemic waged over the cause of bacterial pneumonia, which took place in the 1880's, was one of unusual bitterness, at least on the part of one of the participants engaged therein. Had the arguments been less heated and analysis of the data then at hand more perceptive, events might have followed a course other than that recorded in the ensuing paragraphs.

In 1880, Pasteur[13] and Sternberg[15] recovered from rabbits injected with human saliva what were probably the first strains of pneumococcus to be isolated in the laboratory. At the time, however, the relation of these organisms to lobar pneumonia was far from clear. Despite the fact that bacteria had been seen in the bronchial contents of patients dying of pneumonia by Klebs[12] as early as 1875, their significance remained largely obscure. In the ensuing several years, little significant progress was made aside from the observations of Pasteur and Sternberg.

The first contribution of Carl Friedländer[5] to the etiology of pneumonia appeared in Virchow's Archiv in 1882. Beginning in September, 1881, he had examined the fibrinous exudate of the bronchi and histologic sections of the lungs of eight patients dying of lobar pneumonia. His material was stained with aniline dyes by the Weigert-Koch technique. From his descriptions of the organisms in the pulmonary tissues, it appears altogether probable that Friedländer was looking at the pneumococcus.

Friedländer's second communication[6] on the micrococci of pneumonia appeared on November 15, 1883, and touched off a controversy over the causative agent of pneumonia that was to continue for the next three years. In this paper he reported the study of more than 50 additional cases of pneumonia, in the tissues of nearly all of which bacteria were seen. Those sections from which they were absent were from the lungs of patients dying late in the course of the disease. Friedländer remarked also that the difficulty others had had in recognizing organisms in sections resulted from their being obscured by nuclei and fibrin which stained like bacteria with the techniques usually employed. It is here that he makes the first published reference to the stain of Gram, which facilitated to a hitherto unparalleled degree the recognition of bacteria in histologic sections. Friedländer goes on to describe some of the morphologic properties of the micrococcus of pneumonia, placing especial emphasis on its capsule. Of greater interest, however, is the section devoted to the isolation of the "micrococcus." The bacteriologic work was carried out in collaboration with Dr. Frobenius, who had received his technical training in this field from Koch.

For the growth of organisms, in addition to blood serum, Frobenius prepared a nutrient gelatin which combined meat infusion, peptone and sodium chloride.

The first attempted isolation with this medium was successful. "We isolated from a case of acute pneumonia of the right upper lobe in the stage of grey hepatization (a case with which cirrhosis of the liver was combined but, however, without any complications whatever, even swelling of the spleen was not present) a large number of completely identical cultures, the material for the inoculation of which was taken from three different places of the hepatization."

The cultural properties of the organism isolated are noteworthy. At room temperature, it gave rise in 24 hr to visible growth at the surface of the nutrient gelatin resembling the rounded head of a nail. Similar growth was observed on blood serum, and the organism grew well on potato. Preparations of the micrococcus stained with gentian violet in aniline water were examined and several illustrations accompany the report. In all, the organism is capsulated. Two of the figures show single bacillary forms.

Further attempts to isolate a micrococcus with the properties set forth above were, in the main, unsuccessful. From two additional cases of pneumonia, however, in which both capsulated and noncapsulated micrococci were found, organisms were cultivated which showed a type of colonial growth resembling a flat headed nail with a central depression rather than a round headed nail. This description of colonial morphology suggests that the latter strains were pneumococcus. These two strains were found to be pathogenic in mice but were not subjected, apparently, to extensive study.

Friedländer's investigations of the virulence of his organism in several species of animals are of considerable interest. Rabbits proved to be completely refractory to infection following trans-thoracic inoculation of the lungs. On the other hand, of 11 guinea pigs, 6 succumbed following this type of infection, and mice proved even more susceptible when treated in the same way. Five dogs were inoculated, one of which died, the remainder showing clinical evidence of a mild and transient infection. The findings, in retrospect, resemble more closely those which would be expected to follow inoculation with Friedländer's bacillus, for rabbits are highly susceptible to infection with most types of pneumococcus. Guinea pigs, on the other hand, are often resistant to pneumococci other than type 19[2] but are known to be susceptible to infection with klebsiellas.[1] Friedländer was aware that others had recovered from patients with pneumonia organisms that were virulent for rabbits, but he stated at the time that the materials with which these investigators had worked were not above objection and concluded that the organism he had isolated differed from theirs by virtue of its harmlessness in this laboratory animal.

On April 21, 1884, Fraenkel[3] presented at the Third Congress for Internal Medicine in Berlin the first of a series of communications which was to include important observations establishing the role of pneumococcus in human pneumonia and which contained throughout comments critical of the work of Friedländer. In his initial presentation, Fraenkel described an organism he had isolated from the lung of a 30-year-old man who had succumbed to pneumonia of the right lung. This organism, unlike the one isolated by Friedländer, caused the prompt death of rabbits when inoculated by the same route employed by the latter. Guinea pigs varied in their response, some surviving, others developing pleural and peritoneal effusions from which the injected organism could be recovered. In culture, Fraenkel's coccus failed to produce the nail-head type of growth described by Friedländer. Of two other strains isolated by Fraenkel, however, one differed but little from that described by Friedländer. Fraenkel was unable to decide whether or not the discrepancies observed were the result of differences in the organisms existing prior to their invasion of the human host or of alterations resulting from their residence in the lungs. He took exception, however, to Friedländer's emphasis on the capsule as a unique property of the pneumonia coccus and stated also that the nail-head form of growth was not an essential character of the causative agent of pneumonia. Friedländer responded without rancor and pointed out that, just as he was willing to accept causes of roseola other than typhoid, so was he willing to consider the possibility of more than one agent's ability to cause pneumonia.

Thus the polemic was joined. It is apparent now that at least two bacterial species were probably under study, separable by their cultural characteristics and virulence in laboratory animals. It may be inferred that one was pneumococcus, the other *Klebsiella pneumoniae* or Friedländer's bacillus. Confusion of these two bacterial species today is inconceivable, for they may be distinguished readily by a variety of techniques, none more convenient, perhaps, than by the staining technique of Gram.

And where was Dr. Gram? He was in Friedländer's laboratory where he had devised a technique of staining described briefly by Friedländer in his publication of 1883. Gram published his own report on March 15, 1884,[8] four months after the initial reference to his work. As is already well known to many, Gram devised his technique of staining not for the purpose of distinguishing one group of bacteria from another but to enable bacteria to be seen more readily in stained sections of mammalian tissues. Previously available techniques of staining had made the recognition of bacteria very difficult because nuclei, fibrin, and bacteria manifested similar properties of coloration. By applying a solution of iodine and potassium iodide to sections stained previously with aniline-gentian violet solution and then immersing the sections in alcohol, Gram succeeded in decolorizing the cells of the tissue slices without altering in many instances the blue color of the bacteria therein. He found useful also counterstaining of the tissue with a weak solution of Bismarck brown or Vesuvin.

In his report, Gram made several additional observations, among them the decolorization of the typhoid bacillus when treated by the method outlined. Of greater interest, however, are the findings resulting from the examination of sections of the lungs from fatal cases of lobar pneumonia. In all, Gram examined sections stained by his method from 20 such cases. In 19, the organisms retained the gentian violet (*i.e.*, were gram-positive). In the twentieth case, however, the organisms were decolorized! Of this case, Gram wrote as follows: "One case of croupous pneumonia with capsule-coccus. Here one finds very many cocci which do not all lie in the cells of the exudate. They decolorize very easily in alcohol and, what is more, with and without treatment with iodine. From this case stem a great part of the cultures of Dr. Friedländer. Most of those from animals injected and exposed to infection behave in this fashion (mice, guinea pigs and a dog). Of these, I have investigated some 25 cases. Now and then, the cocci in the experimental animals remain colored after treatment with iodine but then they show no capsule formation; as everyone knows, capsules are always very difficult to demonstrate in cut preparations."

Here then was the key to the problem, but its significance was unappreciated. Although the tinctorial properties of the organism isolated by Friedländer were unique among those of the twenty cases of fatal pneumonia studied by Gram, neither he nor Friedländer gave any sign of having attached any importance to this observation at the time when Gram's paper appeared. Nor, for that matter, did any of the other workers in the field. The potential value of Gram's technique to bacteriology as well as to pathology was to remain unperceived for at least another year.

In the meantime, additional publications relating to the etiology of pneumonia appeared. Of these, perhaps the most extensive in its scope was that of Weichselbaum,[18] who described in 1886 his findings in 129 cases of fatal pneumonia of which 102 were "primary" in character. On the basis of cultural characteristics and of pathogenic properties, he differentiated clearly pneumococcus, to which he gave the nam *Diplococcus pneumoniae*, from Friedländer's bacillus, which he designated *Bacillus pneumoniae*. He recognized that both organisms were capsulated and that the latter could give rise to morphologic variants which resembed cocci. In 94 of the 129 cases studied, Weichselbaum demonstrated pneumococcus microscopically, and he isolated the organism on 54 occasions. *Bacillus pneumoniae* was demonstrated alone or in association with other organisms in 9 instances and was cultivated from 6 of these, from one case together with pneumococcus.

On November 1 of the same year, the following remarks of Friedländer[7] appeared "Weichselbaum found it (*Diplococcus pneumoniae*) 54 times in the pneumonic lung fluid of 83 cases in which cultural techniques were employed; *i.e.*, approximately two thirds of the cases; he holds this coccus identical with the organism found by Fraenkel in seven cases of pneumonia, in lung fluid and in pleural exudate, the description of which appeared several months earlier. From the microscopic state of affairs it is to be added that the coccus is intensely stained by the Gram procedure whereas the organism studied by me is decolorized by the Gram method. . . . From the foregoing investigations it emerges, therefore, that the most frequent organism in pneumonia is a capsulated coccus which was first found by me by microscopic examination (with the attribute of the capsule and the reaction toward the Gram stain), the cultural properties of which meanwhile were established first by Fraenkel and by Weichselbaum. The capsulated bacterium cultivated by me (bacillus of the authors) occurs only in a minority of cases; that it has in fact caused pneumonia in these cases emerges with greater certainty from its presence alone in the lungs and especially from the results of experiments. For it is still, until now, the only known microorganism which evokes, through inhalation, in animals an affection analogous to human lobar pneumonia. The diplococcus studied by the other authors is apparently, for a great number, perhaps for the majority of cases, to be viewed as pathogenic. . . . That an apparently so typical affection as acute pneumonia should be produced by different causes is, as I have already remarked several years ago, to be considered analogous to the causes of acute suppuration. On the other hand, that the same schizomycete should cause two so different affections as rhinoscleroma and pneumonia is likewise most noteworthy."

In this fashion did Friedländer acknowledge the views now held regarding the etiology of pneumonia and at the same time reveal his recognition of the apparent value of the Gram stain. His patience with Fraenkel, however, had begun to wear a little thin, for he added in a footnote: "Of the manifold personal attacks and remonstrances which Fraenkel has directed against me in different places of his work, let them cease. I do not hold them fitting."

It is not altogether clear who was the first to suggest the value of Gram's method of staining in the identification of bacteria. It may have been Ferdinand Hueppe[11] whose book entitled *The Methods of Investigation of Bacteria* was published in 1885. In his discussion of Gram's method he wrote, "A provisional differential diagnosis by means of the microscope becomes possible thereby, for with the Gram method these capsulated cocci* are decolorized whereas the remaining cocci (all?) retain the dye." Similar use of the Gram stain is implied in the text of Huber and Becker[10] published in 1886. Fraenkel was aware of both these texts, as well as of the work of Weichselbaum, when his second paper on the subject of pneumonia that year appeared.[4] He is still berating Friedländer: "Worthy of further mention is the status of microscopic sections of the organs of the different animals with regard to the handling of them by the Gram method of staining. While genuine pneumonia micrococci in sections retain tightly the stain in this procedure, Friedländer's bacillus under identical conditions; *i.e.*, iodine impregnation followed by treatment with alcohol, will be decolorized. In the same way, the rod-shaped organism isolated from the lungs by me behaved." In a footnote he adds: "Herr Weigert had the friendliness to bring first to my attention this peculiar property of Friedländer's bacillus in relation to the Gram method of staining. Thus Gram himself alleged in the original work by him on the method of staining discovered by him that the cocci (one must really call them bacilli) from the case of pneumonia from which a great part of the cultures of Dr. Friedländer stemmed decolorized very easily in alcohol and in fact, with or without treatment with iodine (see Fortschritte der Medicin, 1884, No. 6 S. 189). Hueppe (Die Methoden der Bakterienforschung, Wiesbaden 1885, 1. Aufl. S. 66) says directly that a provisional differential diagnosis of Friedländer's organism from other coccal-like forms becomes possible thereby, that the capsulated cocci stained by the Gram method decolorize and, likewise, in accord with this is the statement in the just published 'pathologisch-histologischen und bakteriologischen Untersuchungsmethoden' by Huber and Becker (Leipsig 1886),

*He is referring to Friedländer's organism.

conf. daselbst S. 89. Herefrom is also to be drawn the conclusion that the Gram method of staining affords us in fact with the potentiality of deciding very directly whether or not in a concrete case of genuine fibrinous pneumonia the organism of Friedländer is present in the exudate."

By 1886, it had been recognized that the typhoid bacillus, cholera vibrio and gonococcus were decolorized by the staining technique of Gram. Of the latter Roux[14] wrote in 1886: "The procedure of Gram employed for the recognition of microorganisms gives no result whatever in gonorrheal pus if the gonococcus is present there alone. One can always recognize their true nature in doubtful cases, however, after having established their presence by staining with gentian violet used alone, by adding successively the liquid of Gram and alcohol. If there is complete disappearance of the cocci, they are indeed those of Neisser; on the other hand, if they retain their violet coloration, one should have doubts as to the gonorrheal nature of the affection and look elsewhere for its true nature."

I am unable to ascertain with certainty when a description of the Gram stain first found its way into a text of bacteriology with intent that it be used for the purpose for which it is employed today. In 1888, Unna[17] published a series of articles on the development of bacterial staining and devoted much space to several aspects of Gram's method. It was recognized at that time that the cocci of pneumonia, pyemia, osteomyelitis, several types of suppuration, and erysipelas retained the aniline dye, whereas the organisms of typhoid, glanders, cholera, and relapsing fever failed to do so. In Thoinot and Masselin's *Précis de Microbie*[16] published in Paris in 1889, the following statement appears: "The method of Gram should always be tried with each given microbe for it furnishes an important diagnostic element according to whether the microbe *takes the Gram or not*" (italics are the authors').

Gram,[9] himself, published only one short note on his method of staining after his initial description of it. It appeared in the proceedings of the 8th Session of the "Congrès Périodique International des Sciences Médicales," which took place in Copenhagen from August 10 to 16, 1884, and contains nothing of additional interest. His subsequent work, until his death in 1935, dealt with other topics.

References

1. Branch, A. 1927 Spontaneous infections of guinea-pigs; pneumococcus, Friedländer bacillus and pseudo-tuberculosis (*Eberthella caviae*). J. Infectious Diseases, 40, 533–548.

2. Finland, M. 1942 Recent advances in the epidemiology of pneumococcal infections. Medicine, 21, 307–344.

3. Fraenkel, A. 1884 Ueber die genuine Pneumonie, Verhandlungen des Congress für innere Medicin. Dritter Congress, 3, 17–31, April 21.

4. Fraenkel, A. 1886 Weitere Beiträge zur Lehre von den Mikrococcen der genuinen fibrinösen Pneumonie. Z. klin. Med., 11 (5/6): 437–458.

5. Friedländer, C. 1882 Ueber die Schizomyceten bei der acuten fibrösen Pneumonie. Virchows Arch. pathol. Anat. u. Physiol., 87 (2): 319–324, Feb. 4.

6. Friedländer, C. 1883 Die Mikrokokken der Pneumonie. Fortschr. Med., 1 (22): 715–733, Nov. 15.

7. Friedländer, C. 1886 Weitere Arbeiten über die Schizomyceten der Pneumonie und der Meningitis. Fortschr. Med., 4 (21): 702–705, Nov. 1.

8. Gram, C. 1884 Ueber die isolierte Färbung der Schizomyceten in Schnitt- und Trockenpräparaten. Fortschr. Med., 2 (6): 185–189, March 15.

9. Gram, C. 1884 Ueber die Färbung der Schizomyceten in Schnittenpräparaten. Congrès périodique international des sciences médicales. 8me Session. Section de pathologie générale et d'anatomie pathologique, p. 116–117. Copenhagen, Aug. 10–16.

10. Huber, K. and Becker, A. 1886 *Die pathologisch-histologischen und bacteriologischen Untersuchungs-Methoden mit einer Darstellung der wichtigsten Bacterien*, p. 87. F. C. W. Vogel, Leipzig.

11. Hueppe, F. 1886 *Die Methoden der Bakterien-Forschung*. (1st ed., C. W. Kreidel. Wiesbaden, 1885, p. 66) 3rd ed., C. W. Kreidel. Wiesbaden 1886, p. 99.

12. Klebs, E. 1875 Beiträge zur Kenntniss der pathogenen Schistomyceten. VII. Die Monadinen. Arch. exptl. Pathol. Pharmakol., 4 (5/6): 409–488, Dec. 10.

13. Pasteur. 1881 Note sur la maladie nouvelle provoquée par la salive d'un enfant mort de la rage. Bull. acad. méd. (Paris), 10, 2e sér.: 94–103, Jan. 25.

    Pasteur, L., Chamberland, and Roux, 1881 Sur une maladie nouvelle provoquée par la salive d'un enfant mort de la rage. Compt. rend., 92 (4): 159–165, Jan.

14. Roux, G. 1886 Sur un procédé technique de diagnose des *gonococci*. Archives générales de médecine, 158 (VIIe sér., vol. 17): 757.

15. Sternberg, G. M. 1881 A fatal form of septicemia in the rabbit produced by the subcutaneous injection of human saliva. Natl. Bd. Health Bull., 2 (44): 781–783, April 30.

16. Thoinot, L. -H., and Masselin, E. -J. 1889 *Précis de microbie*, p. 148. G. Masson, Paris.

17. Unna, P. G. 1888 Die Entwickelung der Bakterienfärbung. Eine historische-kritische Uebersicht (Fortsetzung). Centr. Bakteriol. Parasitenk., 3 (5): 153–158, 1888.

18. Weichselbaum, A. 1886 Ueber die Aetiologie der acuten Lungen- und Rippenfellentzündungen. Medizinische Jahrbücher, 1, 483–554, 1886.

Epilogue

More than twenty years after the foregoing essay was composed, nine letters of Christian Gram came to light.[1] Written in the years 1883 and 1884 to Carl Julius Salomonsen, then a temporary instructor in bacteriology at the University of Copenhagen, they reveal, as the following excerpts show, that Gram had significant reservations about Friedländer's interpretation of their findings. In his letter of January 2, 1884, he wrote: "I have finished my studies on the famous iodine decolorization method which, I assume, will soon be published; however, in this connection there is a difficult point which Friedländer does not quite like. I will have to tamper a little with his work, especially his 'capsules.' It will be somewhat difficult to do that gently. It seems as if there are at least two varieties of pneumonia cocci that look very different. . . ." And again, on June 3, 1884: ". . . . Admittedly there is something 'fishy' about Fr.'s pneumonia cocci. His whole work is very thin, it appears to me. All his cultures and experiments are derived from 1 (one) case which in its pathological anatomy shows great difference from the ordinary pneumonias. Sections of the lungs had not been examined until I found a few small bits; it was that case with cocci (actually they are more like bacteria) which were decolorized after iodine treatment and which occurred lying free [i.e., extracellulary] in the alveoli without much exudate."

From these letters, it is evident that one of the two collaborators was not convinced that the organism advanced by Friedländer as the principal cause of lobar pneumonia in man was indeed the culprit. To those with an interest in history as well as in microbiology and medicine, it is noteworthy that a century elapsed before Gram's personal views of his studies in Friedländer's laboratory were revealed. Despite the latter's gentlemanly defense against Fraenkel's irascible and repeated onslaughts, the scientific base from which Friedländer argued was weak, and his conclusions were to receive later only partial validation.

Reference

Lautrop, H. Christian Gram on the Gram strain in letters to Carl Julius Salomonsen, 1883–1884. ASM News 47:44–49, 1981.

2

The Pneumococcus at Hopkins: Early Portents of Future Developments

Although I cannot recall meeting Dr. Thayer, his name has been well known to me from my boyhood. His photograph hung on the wall of my father's office, one of several of physicians whom he most admired. It is remembered especially for the formality and immaculateness of Dr. Thayer's attire and for the flower worn in the lapel, both hallmarks, as I have gathered from later reading, of Dr. Thayer. The *de facto* recipient of Osler's mantle in many ways, Dr. Thayer was a keen observer of human behavior and an articulate reporter thereof. Through his writings, one perceives readily his scholarship, his gentleness and his sensitivity.[1] Nowhere do these attributes appear more clearly than in his remarks at the dinner marking the presentation of the Thayer Lectureship at the Mayflower Hotel in Washington, D.C., on May 18, 1927, the concluding sentences of which read: "That you my dear master and friend, that you who were my companions and students, and are now my teachers, should make my name an excuse for founding this lectureship on a subject that is so dear to me, is an honour far greater than I deserve. That you should seek to perpetuate my name alongside that of her who was and is the great inspiration of my life, is to do me an honour and to bring me a joy beyond that which I could have conceived—for which I dare not attempt to thank you."[2] In being invited to give one of the Thayer Lectures, I cannot but feel, therefore, both highly complimented and charged with a significant responsibility.

Thayer's writings encompassed a very large part of the subject of internal medicine as was true of the clinician's of his day. His most important contributions in the field of infectious diseases, that area of medicine which has been the focus of most of my professional career, were to the understanding of the malarial fevers[3] and of bacterial endocarditis.[4] He seems to have been little attracted to the subject of respiratory diseases, a topic upon which I shall dwell in much of what follows. Thayer did review the subject of croupous pneumonia in 1899 in Volume 1 of *Progressive Medicine*,[5] and he included a section on pneumococcal endocarditis in his classic monograph on bacterial endocarditis published in 1926 in *The Johns Hopkins Hospital Reports*.[4] Aside from these two publications, however, there is little reference to pneumococcus in his writings. This fact notwithstanding, I thought it might be of interest to look at the role that pneumococcus and pneumococcal disease played in the early days of The Johns Hopkins University and Medical Institutions. One reason for so doing is the approaching centennial of the first isolation of the pneumococcus, just 18 months hence, and a desire to call attention to the little-remembered association of its co-discoverer with The Johns Hopkins University. Other notable figures on the faculty of The Johns Hopkins Medical School in its early days showed a lively interest in pneumococcal infection, and it will be my purpose to review some of their findings and to indicate their relevance to the subsequent and continuing development of our understanding of bacterial disease. Several of these early observations were penetrating indeed and point to problems, some of which remain to challenge those who will confront them in the future.

The First Isolations of the Pneumococcus

The history of the first isolations of the pneumococcus is recounted with great clarity by Welch in a paper entitled, "The Micrococcus Lanceolatus, with Especial Reference to the Etiology of Acute Lobar Pneumonia," which appeared in the *Johns Hopkins Hospital Bulletin* in December 1892: "The micrococcus lanceolatus was discovered by Sternberg in September, 1880, by inoculation of rabbits with his own saliva. It was next found by Pasteur in December, 1880, by inoculating rabbits with the saliva of a child dead of hydrophobia. Pasteur's observations were the first to be made public, being announced at a meeting of the Académie de Médecine in Paris on January 18, 1881. They gave rise to no less than six communications to the same Academy in January, February and March, 1881. Sternberg's first publication on this subject appeared on April 30, 1881."[6]

As indicated in the minutes of the Medical and Chirurgical Faculty of the State of Maryland[7] of its annual meeting held in Baltimore, a verbal announcement of the first isolation of the pneumococcus was made on the campus of

The Johns Hopkins University in Hopkins Hall on April 15, 1881: "The President introduced to the Convention Dr. Sternberg, of the United States Army, who explained in a very interesting manner, 'A Fatal Form of Septicaemia in the Rabbit, produced by the Subcutaneous Injection of Human Saliva.'

"On motion the thanks of the Faculty was tendered Dr. Sternberg for his interesting address, and he was requested to furnish a copy, in writing, for publication in the Transactions."

Sternberg's original report appears in three versions, the first of which was published in the *National Board of Health Bulletin*.[8] The version appearing in the *Transactions of the Medical and Chirurgical Faculty of the State of Maryland* shortly thereafter lacks the last four paragraphs of the original report, for reasons unknown.[9] A third version of the report containing an added section on the morphology of the pneumococcus was published somewhat later in Volume 2 of *Studies from the Biological Laboratory* of The Johns Hopkins University.[10] This last version is of unique historical importance, for it contains the first microphotograph ever made of the pneumococcus.

George Miller Sternberg

Early Years

George Miller Sternberg was an unusual man.[11, 12] The oldest son of a Lutheran minister and the grandson of a doctor of divinity on his maternal side, he was born in Otsego County, New York, in 1838. To help his family, he began teaching school at the age of 16. After several years, he started his medical education; and, on receiving his M.D. degree from the College of Physicians and Surgeons in New York in 1860, he entered the practice of medicine in Elizabeth City, New Jersey. Following the outbreak of the Civil War, he was commissioned an Assistant Surgeon in the United States Army in 1861, marking the start of a medical career with the armed forces that was to continue until his retirement. Sternberg was captured by the Southern forces during the battle of Bull Run but refused to give his parole "not to aid or abet the enemies of the Confederate States of America" and subsequently escaped to rejoin the Northern forces. At the end of the hostilities, he married; but the union was to last less than two years, his wife dying of cholera in Kansas in 1867. Sternberg remarried in 1869; and, accompanied by his second wife, he served in numerous posts throughout the southern and western United States during the next decade, engaged at times in military operations against the

Indians. In 1875, he contracted yellow fever at Fort Barrancas near Pensacola, Florida, and nearly succumbed. This episode marked him as the only member of the Army Medical Corps other than Gorgas to be immune to yellow fever at the outbreak of the Spanish-American War.[13]

Despite the frequent interruptions of regular life occasioned by changes of station and military operations, Sternberg managed to pursue scholarly activities throughout much of his career. He was one of the first in this country or abroad to utilize the technique of photomicrography, described by Mrs. Sternberg in the following terms: "The entire process was so delicate that frequently the jar of a wagon passing on the street would throw an object out of focus and so result in great disappointment."[11] His work on yellow fever is well known to all concerned with the history of that disease. He was one of the early students of bacteriology in this country and published a translation of Magnin's textbook on the subject from French in 1880.[14] Not too dissimilar from the plaintive remarks of contemporary scientists,[15] his comments on the burgeoning of scientific publication, set forth in 1882, have a familiar ring: "The literature on the subject is already enormous, and yearly additions to it seem to grow almost in geometrical progression.

"Note—In the bibliography compiled by Magnin ('The Bacteria,' Little, Brown & Co., Boston, 1880) and added to by myself, but which can be considered by no means complete, the references from 1830–40 are seven; from 1840–50, twelve; from 1850–60, sixty-three; from 1870–80 above three hundred and fifty. In the second volume of the 'Index Catalogue to the Library of the Surgeon-General's Office,' just published, four closely printed pages are required for references relating to 'Charbon' alone."[16]

Initial Studies of the Pneumococcus

Although the pneumococcus was probably seen first by Klebs in 1875 in the bronchial contents of patients dying of pneumonia,[17] there can be little doubt that Sternberg was the first to isolate the organism and to grow it *in vitro*. In 1880, he was sent to New Orleans to investigate the cause of malarial fever. What followed is best expressed, perhaps, in Sternberg's own words, published on April 30, 1881:

In a report (not yet published) made to the National Board of Health in February last, I have given a detailed account of certain experiments, made in the first instance as a check upon experiments relating to the so-called *Bacillus malariae* of Klebs and

Tommasi-Crudeli, which show that my own saliva has remarkable virulent properties when injected into the subcutaneous tissue of a rabbit. Further experiments, made in the biological laboratory of the Johns Hopkins University, have fully confirmed the results heretofore obtained, and the object of the present report is to place upon the record these last experiments which are of special interest just now because of the announcement by Pasteur of "*a new disease*," produced in rabbits by the subcutaneous injection of the saliva of an infant which died of hydrophobia in one of the hospitals of Paris (Comptes Rendus Ac. d. sc. 1881, xcii, p 159).

I have demonstrated by repeated experiments that my saliva in doses of $1.25c^3$ to $1.75c^3$ (see note 1) injected into the subcutaneous connective tissue of a rabbit, infallibly produces death within forty-eight hours.

Query. Does the saliva of other individuals injected in the same manner produce similar results?

Answer. The saliva of four students, residents of Baltimore (in March), gave negative results; eleven rabbits injected with saliva of six individuals in Philadelphia (in January) gave eight deaths and three negative results; . . . [8]

Sternberg went on to describe his studies of the virulence of human saliva in other animal species, the clinical and pathological changes observed in injected rabbits and the presence in their blood of an "immense number of micrococci, usually joined in pairs and having a diameter of 0.5μ." By filtration of saliva and of the sera of infected rabbits, he demonstrated the particulate nature of the infectious agent and showed also that its virulence was destroyed by boiling or by the addition of carbolic acid to saliva. He succeeded in growing the organism in bouillon made from rabbit flesh and in fulfilling Koch's postulates by reproducing illness in animals inoculated with the cultured bacteria.

It is noteworthy that Sternberg became aware so promptly of Pasteur's findings which were presented to the French Academy on January 26, 1881, only three months before the publication of Sternberg's report in this country. He had spent the first part of that year working in the Department of Medicine at the University of Pennsylvania before coming to Baltimore, where he became a Fellow by Courtesy of The Johns Hopkins University. As noted in the President's report for the academic year 1880–1881: "The persons below have been resident at the University for purposes of scientific and literary work during the whole or a considerable part of the academic year, and by courtesy have been accorded the usual privileges of Fellow." [18]

The version of Sternberg's initial report published in the *Studies from the Biological Laboratory* of The Johns Hopkins University [10] contained a section on morphology not included in the one published in the *National Board of*

Health Bulletin.[8] In it, one finds reference to Sternberg's mistaken notion that Pasteur had thought originally the pneumococcus to have been the cause of rabies.

Since writing the report published in "*The Bulletin*" of April 30th, my attention has been called to the fact that M. Vulpian has arrived at similar results (Bull. de l'Acad. de Med., March 29, 1881); and I infer that Pasteur has somewhat changed his opinion as to the nature of the "new disease" described by him in his communication to the French Academy (made January 26th), from the following remark of Chauveau, which I find in his recent address, as President of the French Association for Advancement of Science. (Revue Scientifique, April 16th, 1881). He says:

"For a moment we had hoped that Pasteur had determined thus" (by artificial cultivation) "the virus of hydrophobia, *but he tells us himself that he has only cultivated a new septic agent.*"

In this section, Sternberg describes also the capsule of the pneumococcus, noting that its presence had been observed by Pasteur as well: "The most striking morphological difference between the micrococcus as shown in Figures 2, 3 and 4, and in Figure 1, is the aureole which surrounds the well-defined dark central portion in the latter figure.

"Pasteur says of this appearance: 'This organism is sometimes so small that it may escape a superficial observation. . . . It is an extremely short rod, a little compressed toward the middle resembling a figure 8. . . . *Each of these little particles is surrounded at a certain focus with a sort of aureole which corresponds perhaps to a material substance.*'"

It is clear from these remarks that each of the first two microbiologists to isolate the pneumococcus recognized the capsule as one of its attributes.

Immunogenic Properties of Saliva

Sternberg published a number of additional reports in 1882 on the organism in human saliva causing septicemia in the rabbit, several of which contain intimations of important attributes of the pneumococcus to be delineated later by others. As early as 1878, he had begun a series of studies on disinfectants which brought him the Lomb Prize in 1886. The techniques of these investigations were applied to the newly discovered bacterium. In two reports, one in *Studies from the Biological Laboratory* of The Johns Hopkins University [19] and a second published in the *American Journal of the Medical Sciences*,[20] there are suggestions of the immunogenic properties of the organism as indicated by the following quotation from the latter:

> The number of experiments upon which this announcement rests I am not able to give at the present moment, as my detailed report of these experiments is in the hands of the National Board of Health and I have not retained a copy at hand. I think, however, that I am quite safe in saying that I have repeated the experiment at least twenty-five times with my own saliva. But experiments made subsequently to the writing of the above quotation from my original report make it necessary for me to slightly qualify the language of this. I can no longer say *infallibly* produces death, as in several instances death has not occurred in rabbits which have been previously injected with saliva mixed with certain substances—alcohol, quinine—which when added to it in a certain proportion, prevent the usual fatal results, but do not prevent an impression being made by the mixed injections which seems subsequently to protect the animal from the lethal effects of injections of saliva alone.

It would appear that the results following the injection of saliva containing pneumococci and treated with a disinfectant are precisely those to be expected to ensue after successful vaccination.

The same year, Claxton, in Philadelphia, repeated several of the studies described earlier.[21] "My experiments were performed in great part," he wrote, "as a check on those of Sternberg." Sternberg, meanwhile, had left Baltimore for San Francisco, where he continued his observations, several of which were reported in the *Philadelphia Medical Times*,[22,23] one with the following introductory remarks: "I should be very sorry to dose the readers of the *Medical Times* with saliva *ad nauseum*; but having experimental data to record, I thought it best to publish at once while the subject is still fresh in the minds of the readers of this journal from a perusal of Dr. Claxton's paper and my own."[23]

By repeated transfer of the pneumococcus through sequential broth cultures interrupted periodically by animal passage, Sternberg calculated that he had diluted the original inoculum 1,679,611,600,000,000 times without impairing its virulence. ". . . . Yet some very conservative physicians still claim that the invading parasite is without import, a mere epi-phenomenon, while the infinitesimal portion of the hypothetical chemical virus is credited with the malignant potency. Truly, such a belief requires a faith equal to that of a conscientious homoeopath. By the way, what will become of homoeopathy if the germ theory becomes firmly established, and all infectious diseases are shown to be due to parasitic micro-organisms? If the main end of therapeutics is to kill germs, the doctrine of *similia similibus* can scarcely control the medical practice of the future."[23]

Sternberg made one additional, possibly prophetic, observation in this series of reports: "How it happens that the micrococcus in one man's mouth possesses just the proper degree of vital activity to kill a rabbit in two days, while that from another man's mouth kills in four days and that from another does not kill at all, is a most interesting question and one worthy of the attention of future investigations."[22] One can only speculate regarding the role played in these experiments by different pneumococcal capsular types, the recognition of which was not to take place for another 28 years.[24]

Coincident with the publication of Sternberg's last paper to be entitled "Virulence of Normal Human Saliva," there appeared in the *Philadelphia Medical Times* the following editorial headed: "Johns Hopkins Hospital":

It is stated in the *Maryland Medical Journal* that the trustees of the Johns Hopkins University propose opening that institution next autumn. The buildings, with the exception of the laundry, are all under roof, one million three hundred thousand dollars having been spent upon them. In none of them has any inside work been done, other than flooring, staircases, and heating apparatus, and to finish during the coming summer will require active work. The buildings, when complete, will, in our opinion, be the finest of the kind in the world. The medical school may well be in operation two years before the hospital is in full activity. The course of instruction is to be extended over four years, and the students will not be ready for practical bedside study until their third year. We are not in the secrets of the trustees of the University, but it is plain that the time is approaching when the medical faculty must be appointed. For the honor of our country, but especially for the good of the race, we trust the great opportunities now afforded will be wisely embraced. With proper selections, Johns Hopkins University and Medical School may become a great centre of light and progress in the science and practice of medicine. The American intellect is equal to any in the world: what is needed is opportunity.[25]

Prophetic words!

The Association of Pneumococcus With Pneumonia

Sternberg returned to Baltimore in 1884, and renewed his ties with Hopkins, working part of the time in the Pathological Laboratory with Welch, again with the title of Fellow by Courtesy, The Johns Hopkins University, which he held until 1890, when he was transferred once more to San Francisco. Much had happened in the interval betwen Sternberg's two sojourns in the Monumental City. In 1880, Koch[26] and Eberth,[27] independently, had seen what were almost certainly pneumococci in the lungs and cerebrospinal fluids of patients with pneumonia and meningitis. Friedländer published his first reports on the etiology of pneumonia in 1882[28] and 1883[29] and was engaged in a polemic with Fraenkel in 1884[30] over the bacterial cause of this infection. Of especial interest are the two seldom cited brief reports of Günther[31] and of Leyden,[32] presented to the Society for Internal Medicine of Berlin on November 20, 1882. On May 3 of the same year, Günther had performed a lung puncture with a Pravaz'sch syringe of the right lower lobe of a 48-year-old man with pneumonia. At a depth of 3 cm he obtained a few drops of cloudy sanguino-purulent fluid, which on microscopic examination showed lymphoid cells, red blood corpuscles and numerous diplococci both in unstained and stained preparations. The patient died five hours following the procedure and, at autopsy, was found to have pleural adhesions at the site of the puncture, assuring thereby that the aspirated material had come from the lung and not from the pleural cavity. Leyden, who preceded Günther on the program, described a similar case: "I have now 10 days ago made a puncture in a patient with pneumonia with a Pravaz'sch syringe and could demonstrate in the blood withdrawn with the familiar dry method through staining with methylene blue these organisms. The drawings which I have had made I will now pass around. They are for the most part diplococci and indeed most significantly of oval shape. . . . I will note additionally that I had already made a puncture the day before which had not given clear results which, however, encouraged me to repeat the puncture."

It is of interest that both Friedländer and Fraenkel were present at this meeting and commented upon the presentations. The remark of Fraenkel is of especial interest: "According to the drawing which Herr Günther has laid before us, it appears as if the cocci are surrounded by an unstained capsule."

Sternberg was evidently aware of a number of these European publications. In 1885, he published a paper entitled "The Pneumonia-coccus of Friedländer (*Micrococcus Pasteuri*, Sternberg),"[33,34] which had been read before the Pathological Society of Philadelphia in April of that year. This report marks the first linking by Sternberg of the organism isolated from his own saliva with the cause of pneumonia. In it, he has confused what has now come to be known as klebsiella with pneumococcus and has again alluded to his mistaken impression that Pasteur had thought originally the pneumococcus to be the cause of rabies. It is a tribute to Sternberg's generosity of spirit, however, that although he had isolated the pneumococcus three months before Pasteur, he recognized the latter's priority of publication and named the organism of sputum septicemia "*Micrococcus Pasteuri*, Sternberg."

In 1886, Sternberg visited Berlin and volunteered to demonstrate the organism he had discovered in his own saliva to Robert Koch. The story is described by Mrs. Sternberg: "On his return from the laboratory he was somewhat absorbed in thought and when, early the next morning, I asked him the reason for his anxious expression, he confided to me the promise made on the preceding day. 'How dreadful I would feel,' he said, 'if I have lost that germ in the meantime from my mouth and could not demonstrate a thing I have written and talked so much about.' But when the demonstration was attempted in Dr. Koch's laboratory, it was most satisfactory, and a clean proof was recorded in favor of Sternberg's previous claim."[11]

By 1889, the role of the pneumococcus as the chief cause of lobar pneumonia had been fully established. The history of the preceding nine years is reviewed by Sternberg in a communication entitled "The Etiology of Croupous Pneumonia,"[35] and his own experimental findings are set in this context. A paper bearing the same title which appeared in the *National Medical Review* of December 1897 contains one additional noteworthy comment of his: "I object to the name 'diplococcus pneumoniae' because this micrococcus in certain culture media forms longer or shorter chains and it is in fact a streptococcus."[36] Approximately 80 years were to elapse before American bacteriologists were to adopt this view, the accepted scientific name of pneumococcus in this country having been changed only recently to "*Streptococcus pneumoniae*."[37]

Sternberg's formal affiliation with The Johns Hopkins University terminated in 1890 although he continued his associations with a number of his colleagues in Baltimore. Both Osler and Welch attended and spoke at the dinner held in New York in June 1902, on the occasion of his retirement as Surgeon General from the Army. Sternberg died in Washington, D.C., on November 3, 1915. His epitaph was written by Welch: "Pioneer American Bacteriologist: Distinguished by his studies of the causation and prevention of infectious diseases, by his discovery of the microorganism of pneumonia, and scientific investigations of yellow fever, which paved the way for the experimental demonstration of the mode of transmission of that pestilence. Veteran of three wars, brevetted for bravery in action in the Civil War and the Nez Percés War. Served as Surgeon General of the U.S. Army for a period of nine years, including the Spanish War. Founder of the Army Medical School. Scientist, author and philanthropist. M.D., L.L.D."[11]

Here was a Fellow by Courtesy of whom Hopkins can indeed be proud, and whose manifold accomplishments seem well worth recalling as the centennial of his isolation of the pneumococcus approaches.

Contributions of Welch and of Osler

As indicated earlier, Welch, in whose laboratory Sternberg had worked, took an active interest in the evolving knowledge of the pneumococcus and its role as a human pathogen. In Volume 1 of *The Johns Hopkins Hospital Bulletin*, his "Remarks on the Diplococcus pneumoniae at the meeting of the Johns Hopkins Hospital Medical Society of February 17th, 1890," attended by 36 members, are reported.[38] "The history of our knowledge of this organism from its discovery by Sternberg in September, 1880, up to the present time and the results and conclusions reached by the various investigators of its relation to croupous pneumonia were briefly reviewed. The frequent presence of the pneumococcus in the saliva of healthy persons is upon the whole an assistance to us in the explanation of the various factors concerned in the causation of croupous pneumonia." An earlier note in the same volume of the *Bulletin* notes that Welch exhibited and described cultures from cases of acute croupous pneumonia.[39] Welch wrote two additional and detailed accounts of the pneumococcus, one serving as his Presidential Address to the Medical and Chirurgical Faculty of the State of Maryland, given to an audience of approximately 200 physicians at the Hall of the Faculty at St. Paul and Saratoga Streets on April 26th, 1892[40]; the other, in Volume 3 of *The Johns Hopkins Hospital Bulletin*, the first of a promised series of reports "based upon my lectures on the causation of acute lobar pneumonia, delivered at the Johns Hopkins Hospital in January, February and March, 1892, and upon the presidential address before the Medical and Chirurgical Faculty of the State of Maryland in April, 1892."[6] Subtitled "First Article," it was unfortunately the only one of the projected series to be published. As observed in a footnote in Volume 2 of the Papers and Addresses by William H. Welch: "[This article is the first installment of a series of papers, the latter, however, never having been published]."[41] The reprint does contain, fortunately, the list of references cited in the article which appeared in the *Bulletin* but which are lacking from this journal in which the article was printed originally. Welch's treatment of his subject is encyclopedic, and his failure to publish the additional material is a cause for regret.

Osler's early observations on pneumococcal infection appear to have stemmed from his interest in bacterial endocarditis. His paper, "Infectious (so-called Ulcerative) Endocarditis," published in 1881 while he was still at McGill University, calls attention to the frequent association of primary infectious endocarditis with pneumonia.[42] This observation is dilated upon in the Gulstonian Lectures of 1885 when there was still active debate as to the cause of lobar pneumonia. Osler's comments at the time are of interest:

In pneumonia, micrococci undoubtedly abound in exudation in the air cells and their mode of growth in gelatine is peculiar, but the numerous experiments on artificial production are not yet conclusive. The evidence is accumulating which places pneumonia among the infective disorders and it certainly is a seductive view to take of its pathology to regard the local pulmonary lesion as excited by the growth of micrococci in the air cells, and the various consecutive inflammations—the endocarditis and pericarditis, the pleurisy, the meningitis, the membranous gastritis or colitis—as due to the penetration of the organisms to deeper parts, and their local development under conditions dependent on the state of the tissues. The processes are all of the character described as croupous, and have as a common feature the presence of micrococci in a coagulable exudation. We have still, however, to settle the identity of the organisms of the air cells with those of the consecutive inflammations, but we may reasonably hope ere long to have some positive data from investigations in this disease which, more than any other, offers favourable opportunities for the solution of these problems.[43]

Osler's writings on pneumonia, and especially his changing philosophic views on the role of that disease, set forth in successive editions of his famous textbook of medicine, are widely known and often quoted. Early in his tenure at Hopkins, Osler established a durable tradition of reviewing annually the cases of pneumonia admitted to the Johns Hopkins Hospital, one that was to yield much useful clinical information over the years. In 1897, he wrote:

For the past eight weeks, we have been studying together the prevalent acute diseases—malaria and typhoid fever; and now the picture begins to change, and the presence in the wards of several cases reminds us that the pneumonia season is at hand. We shall begin today a systematic study of this the most important acute affection you will be called upon to treat—a disease with manifestations perhaps less multiform than typhoid fever or malaria but one infinitely more dangerous and much less under our control. As our aim is to make this a school of practical medicine, I dispense as far as possible with all theoretical and didactic considerations and make the cases teach the lessons of the disease. In the ward classes you will see (as far as is possible) and have notes of every case of pneumonia admitted this session, and I have asked one of your number to be Recorder, and fill up week by week on the blackboard a tabular list, so that you can, as we say, "keep track" of them.[44]

One of the early fruits of Osler's practice was a series of reports reviewing many of the aspects of pneumonia and its complications, based upon a 16-year experience with the disease at The Johns Hopkins Hospital starting in 1889, and published in Volume 15 of *The Johns Hopkins Hospital Reports*. There are 11 papers in all, touching on almost every aspect of the illness.

Recovery From Pneumococcal Pneumonia: The Crisis

Observations on the termination of lobar pneumonia prior to the avail-ability of either serum or antimicrobial therapy are of especial interest to the contemporary student of infectious disease. In view of the emphasis in text-books on the crisis as the characteristic mode of recovery from pneumococcal pneumonia, the frequency of its occurrence among those recovering in the se-ries reported, 37.1%, seems strikingly low.[45,46] That it is an event which may still be observed occasionally in the era of antimicrobial therapy, I have learned painfully from first-hand experience.

Nineteen hundred forty-nine was the year marking the introduction of chlor-tetracycline (Aureomycin®, Lederle), and it was available then for clinical in-vestigation on the Osler Medical Service. It was also the year that I served as the Osler resident. One of the resident's pleasant duties at Christmas time was to escort the choir from one of the local churches through the hospital wards where its members sang carols on Christmas Eve to cheer those unable to be at home for the holiday. Engaged in this activity, I got a call from the Obstetrical Service to see a 19-year-old female with cough and high fever, in her eighth month of pregnancy. It took no special skill to discover that she had lobar pneumonia involving her right lower lobe with all the classical signs of con-solidation. I obtained a blood culture and a sample of her sputum in which I was able to identify without difficulty large numbers of pneumococcus type 8 by the direct quellung reaction. As an aside, one of the benefits of the Osler internship before World War II was a month's experience in the bacteriological laboratory doing all the cultures for the service. It taught one, among other things, what cultures and how many were useful to obtain and gave one also a critique of such a laboratory, one useful in evaluating others on which one might have later to depend. The diagnosis of the patient's illness being clear on this occasion, I convinced myself at the time that pregnancy was not an illness and that I could safely determine the efficacy of Aureomycin® in the treatment of her pneumonia. I returned to the Obstetrical Service, wrote orders for the drug and for her to be placed in an oxygen tent and went back to the choir. After the singers had departed, there were several other consultations; and I got to bed in Osler's quarters at quite a late hour. Early Christmas morn, the student nurses awakened me, singing carols around the statue in the hospital's foyer. In the cold light of dawn, I began to have second thoughts about the wisdom of my therapeutic decision of the previous night. I dressed and went directly to the Obstetrical Service to see the patient. Well, I couldn't have had a nicer Christmas present. Her temperature had fallen from 104°F to 98°F; she wanted to get out of the oxygen tent and also was demanding breakfast! Feeling very pleased indeed, I went over to the Osler wards and started my daily rounds. An hour later, I was paged by George W. Corner, Jr., then the resident in Obstetrics. "Good morning, George," said I, "Merry Christmas!" "Bob," he replied, "do you remember that girl with pneumonia you saw last night?" "Of course," I said. "Well," he said, "something terrible has happened." My heart sank. "What's happened?" I asked. "You know that girl with pneumonia?" he queried again. "Yes," I said, "and if you don't tell me what is the matter, I'm coming over and punch you in the nose. What's happened?" "Well, guess what," said George, "we just made her bed and we found every one of those capsules you left for her under her pillow!" The patient had had a natural crisis and had clearly got well without any help from medication. Needless to state, I was enormously relieved though no little deflated by what had occurred. The experience taught me, first-hand, a lesson in therapeutics I have never forgotten and brought home clearly the portent of my father's comment (I do not know if it originated with him) that most patients get well in spite of doctors.

The Pathogenesis of Pneumococcal Bacteremia

Other early studies, including those of pneumococcal bacteremia and of extrapulmonary pneumococcal infection in the absence of pneumonia, are of considerable interest as they relate to the pathogenesis of bacteremia caused by this organism. Pneumococcal bacteremia was demonstrated first probably by Friedländer in 1884* although the identity of the organism he isolated by cupping from 1 of 6 patients with pneumonia is not established with certainty.[47] The occurrence of bacteremia as a complication of pneumonia is cited by Futcher in a paper entitled "The Blood in Pneumonia" published in the *National Medical Review* in 1897.[48] In it, Futcher observes: "Bacteriological examination of the blood in pneumonia can never be expected to come into general use for diagnostic purposes. . . . Clinical experience has shown that the prognosis in those cases where the organism gets into the general circulation is extremely bad."

In 1902, Rufus Cole, then an Assistant Resident Physician and Instructor in

*See Chapter 5, p. 70 and rf. 15, p. 76.

Medicine at Hopkins and later Director of the Hospital of the Rockefeller Institute, reviewed the blood cultures of 30 patients on Osler's service in the winter of 1900–1901, 29 of whom had lobar pneumonia.[49] All nine patients with bacteremia succumbed whereas only four of 21 lacking bacteremia died. One patient with meningitis and arthritis and lacking pneumonia is described by him in greater detail in the same issue of *The Johns Hopkins Hospital Bulletin*.[50] Aside from findings of slight terminal bronchopneumonia, this patient showed no evidence at autopsy of having had focal pneumococcal infection to account for his bacteremia.

Further evidence for the occurrence of focal pneumococcal infection in the absence of lobar pneumonia appears in several of the reviews of this disease and its complications in the volume of *The Johns Hopkins Hospital Reports* cited earlier. Seven of 25 cases of pneumococcal meningitis described by Hanes were unassociated with pneumonia and, in three of the seven, no primary focus of infection could be found, even in the two who were autopsied.[51] In the remaining four patients, meningeal infection appeared to be the sequel to focal infection of the paranasal sinuses.

Howard, in a report of three cases of pneumococcal arthritis, describes one occurring in a 55-year-old black male in the absence of lobar pneumonia.[52] In his discussion of non-pneumonic pneumococcal arthritis, he cites the observation of Herzog that such infection is relatively and absolutely more common in infancy and childhood than in adult life, in which it is a rarity.[53] "Thus Herzog found in 28 cases of infants under 2 years, 11 cases with no *previous* pneumonia (39.9%), in 8 children between 2 and 14 years, 5 cases with no previous pneumonia (62.5%), while in 55 adults there were only 4 cases without a previous pneumonia."

These early observations of pneumococcal infections of serous cavities of humans in the absence of demonstrable focal infection of the upper or lower respiratory tract raise interesting questions regarding their pathogenesis. In experimental animals, following intrapulmonary instillation of pneumococci, bacteremia appears to be the sequel to spread of the organisms via the pulmonary lymphatic vessels to the hilar lymph nodes, where, if their progress is not checked, they enter the thoracic duct via the efferent lymphatic vessels of the mediastinal lymph glands. Bacteremia in such an experimental model does not occur in the absence of infection of the thoracic duct lymph.[54] Suggestive pathological evidence for the spread of pneumococci via the lymphatic channels to the blood of man was described by Wandel in 1903,[55] and the histopathology of bacterial lymphadenitis has been carefully elucidated by Smith and Wood.[56,57] A second recognized pathway for the development of pneumococcal bacteremia has been that involving extension of a focal infection of the upper respiratory tract to the subarachnoid space and passage of the organisms through the arachnoid villi into the venous sinuses draining the meninges.[58] How frequently pneumococci cause bacteremia as a sequel to sinusitis or otitis media is difficult to assess because of the paucity of data relating to this subject.

Unlike meningococci and *Haemophilus influenzae* type b, which are thought to produce illness as a sequel to bacteremia developing in asymptomatic as well as in symptomatic nasopharyngeal carriers of these organisms, pneumococci have not been thought, until recently, to cause infection under comparable circumstances. In his monograph entitled "The Biology of Pneumococcus," White wrote as follows: "From time to time bacteriologists have alleged that virulent pneumococci as well as streptococci and other pathogens are to be found in the circulating blood of healthy persons as well as those ill with affections to which these organisms are not related. The validity of the claims is always highly questionable, and it is problematical if Pneumococcus invades the circulatory system unless a specific focus of infection exists at some point in the body."[59] Observations made in the last 12 years, however, suggest that pneumococcal bacteremia in man may arise in a fashion analogous to that observed following colonization of the upper respiratory tract with other capsulated bacterial pathogens.

Rake described bacteremia in mice inoculated intranasally with pneumococci, bacteremia which was observed within minutes of placing organisms on the nasal mucous membrane.[60] Schulz and his coworkers, in studies of the lymphatic circulation of the rabbit, showed that pneumococci could be isolated from the lymphatic vessels of the neck following the nasal instillation of type III pneumococci and that the appearance of organisms in the lymph antedated their appearance in the blood.[54] In these animals, the trachea was cannulated and the esophagus tied to prevent the ingress of pneumococci into the systemic or lymphatic circulation from the lower respiratory or gastrointestinal tract. Pretreatment of the animals with type-specific antiserum reduced the likelihood of pneumococci being isolated from the cervical lymphatic vessels and also from the circulation. Although comparable findings in man are not available, several recent clinical observations are in accord with the experimental ones.

In 1967, Belsey reported three cases of pneumococcal bacteremia in children aged 10 to 21 months, in one of whom no focus of infection could be found.[61] Since the appearance of this report, the occurrence of pneumococcal bacteremia in febrile infants and children often lacking focal signs of infection has been documented repeatedly in clinics where blood cultures are obtained routinely from febrile patients.[62-66] Pneumococcus has been the organism isolated most often from the blood of such patients and has been recovered with a frequency of about 2.5%.[62] Most of these bacteremias have been observed in children aged 7 to 24 months. An interesting feature of these infections is the fact that by the time the bacteremia was identified, the patient had frequently recovered from his illness and without the benefit of antimicrobial therapy. In one quarter to one half of the patients observed in different studies, no local site of infection in either the upper or lower respiratory tract could be identified at either the initial or the follow-up examination. Several patients, including both those who had or who had not been given antimicrobial therapy, developed metastatic infection, notably pneumococcal meningitis.

That findings comparable to those observed in pediatric populations have not been reported heretofore in adults may result from the fact that levels of antibody to pneumococci and to other bacteria in man tend to increase with maturation. In a study of antibodies to several pneumococcal capsular types prior to colonization with these types of family members of different ages, levels of antibodies were approximately threefold higher in children aged 6 to 16 years than they were in younger children; and in individuals over 16 years of age, they tended to be tenfold higher than in those aged 6 to 16 years.[67] In addition, the incidence of bacteremia in early life is highest between the ages of 7 and 12 months, following the disappearance of placentally transferred maternal antibody and prior to the infant's development of its own antibody.[64] These findings are consistent with the experimental data from rabbits in which the presence of antibody impeded lymphatic spread of organisms from the upper respiratory tract and reduced the incidence of bacteremia.

In light of the foregoing observations, findings in the recent pneumococcal vaccine trials carried out in populations of gold mining novices in South Africa are of interest. Over a four-year period in a population of 12,000 young adult males, a third of whom received one or another of two formulations of polyvalent pneumococcal vaccine, 217 bacteremic infections were observed. Among 152 individuals who had pneumococcal bacteremia and were x-rayed, 15 had normal postero-anterior films of the chest. Of these, approximately half had physical findings compatible with an infection of the lower respiratory tract. In addition, there were 15 individuals admitted to hospital with fever and headache but lacking both symptoms and signs of respiratory infection. Blood cultures were otained from these men because their temperatures equaled or exceeded 101°F at some time during their hospitalization, and all cultures contained pneumococci of one of four types, types 12, 25, 45 or 46. None of these individuals was given any form of antimicrobial therapy, and all but one, who was readmitted a day after discharge with lobar pneumonia, remained well and returned to work. This group of patients represents one strikingly similar to those pediatric groups with pneumococcal bacteremia described in recent years. Unfortunately sera are not available from these individuals and from young children of the same population to permit a determination of whether or not antibodies to pneumococcal capsular polysaccharides were comparably low in both groups. One might surmise that they were in view of both the available experimental laboratory and clinical findings.

It would appear likely, therefore, that pneumococcal bacteremia may arise in one of three ways: as a sequal to focal infection of the upper respiratory tract with or without involvement of the meninges; as a sequel to pneumonia and to the failure of the host's defensive mechanisms to check the spread of the infection in the lung and mediastinal lymph nodes; and, finally, as a result of spread to the systemic circulation via the cervical lymphatics as a sequel to colonization, but in the absence of overt infection of the nasopharynx. Such a mechanism would be similar to that thought to be the principal route of infection in meningococcemia and in such systemic infections as meningitis and arthritis caused by *H. influenzae* type b at times in the absence of overt respiratory infection. Such a route of infection in the individual lacking antibody to a given pneumococcal polysaccharide and afflicted with pneumococcal arthritis, meningitis, peritonitis or endocarditis in the absence of symptoms or signs of upper or lower respiratory infection would seem reasonable to hypothesize. This mode of pathogenesis is altogether in accord with recent observations in pediatric populations and with the findings in adults from Malawi and Mozambique. It would provide an explanation also for some clinical observations made at The Johns Hopkins Hospital three quarters of a century ago, an era in which many fundamental observations on infectious disease were being made by investigators with remarkably keen perceptions.

Toxemia of Pneumococcal Infection: A Major Unsolved Problem

Despite many advances since those earlier days, unsolved problems remain, none more important, perhaps, than the origin of the toxemia of pneumococcal infection, so well described in the following passage by Osler:

The toxemia is the important element in the disorder to which in the majority of cases the degree of pyrexia and the consolidation are entirely subsidiary. The poisonous factors may develop early and cause from the outset severe cerebral symptoms and they are not necessarily proportionate to the degree of lung involved. There may be severe and fatal toxemia with consolidation of only one-half a lobe, while the patient with complete solidification of one lobe or of a whole lung may from beginning to close of the attack have no *delirium* . . .

Very large areas of the breathing surface may be cut off without disturbing the cardiorespiratory mechanism. In no way is this more strikingly shown than by the condition of the patient after the crisis. On one day with a lung consolidated from apex to base, the respirations from 60 to 65 and the temperature between 104° and 105°, the patient may seem in truly desperate condition, and it would appear rational to attribute the urgent dyspnoea and the slight cyanosis to the mechanical interference with the exchange of gases in the lungs. But on the following day, dyspnoea and cyanosis may have disappeared, the temperature is normal and the pulse rate greatly lessened, and yet the physical condition of the lungs remains unchanged. We witness no more striking phenomenon than this in the whole range of clinical work and its lesson is of prime importance in this very question, showing that the fever and the toxins rather than the solid exudate are the essential agents in causing cardiorespiratory symptoms. . . .

The toxemia outweighs all other elements in the prognosis of pneumonia; to it (the gradual failure of strength or more rarely in a sudden death, as here given) is due in great part the terrible mortality from this common disease and unhappily against it we have as yet no reliable measures at our disposal.[68]

Unfortunately, we seem no closer to a solution of this problem than when these words were written in 1897. Its elucidation remains a challenge for the future.

To have been invited to give this lecture has prompted me to learn more of the legacy of Dr. Thayer and his contemporaries, and this has been my reward. To quote Cotton Mather from Thayer's essay on Mather's rules of health: "'Tis a Trespass on the Rules of Prudence never to know when to have done. Wherefore, I have done!"[69]

References

1. Hunley, E. S.: Bibliography of the writings of Dr. William S. Thayer. Bull. Instit. Hist. Med.: 4: 751–781, 1936.

2. Thayer, W. S.: Remarks on the presentation of the Thayer Lectureship. Bull. Johns Hopkins Hosp. 41: 7–10, 1927.

3. Thayer, W. S.: Lectures on the Malarial Fevers. New York: D. Appleton & Co., 1897.

4. Thayer, W. S.: Studies on bacterial (infective) endocarditis. Johns Hopkins Hosp. Rep. 22: 1–185, 1926.

5. Thayer, W. S.: Infectious disease including croupous pneumonia. Prog. Med. 1: 281–343, 1899.

6. Welch, W. H.: The Micrococcus lanceolatus, with especial reference to the etiology of acute lobar pneumonia. Johns Hopkins Hosp. Bull. 3: 125–139, 1892.

7. Minutes of the Medical and Chirurgical Faculty of the State of Maryland. Tr. Med. Chir. Fac. State of Md. 83: 17, 1881.

8. Sternberg, G. M.: A fatal form of septicaemia in the rabbit, produced by subcutaneous injection of human saliva. An experimental research. Natl. Bd. of Health Bull. 2: 781–783, 1881.

9. Sternberg, G. M.: A fatal form of septicaemia in the rabbit, produced by the subcutaneous injection of human saliva. An experimental research. Tr. Med. Chir. Fac. State of Md. 83: 210–219, 1881.

10. Sternberg, G. M.: A fatal form of septicaemia in the rabbit, produced by the subcutaneous injection of human saliva. Studies from the Biol. Lab. of the Johns Hopkins Univ. 2: 183–200, 1882.

11. Sternberg, M. L.: George Miller Sternberg, A Biography. Chicago: American Medical Assn., 1920.

12. Gibson, J. M.: Soldier in White. The Life of General George Miller Sternberg. Durham: Duke Univ. Press, 1958.

13. Memorial: General William Crawford Gorgas. Trans. Am. Climat. Clin. Assn. 37: xxi–xxv, 1921.

14. Magnin, A.: The Bacteria. Translated by G. M. Sternberg. Boston: Little, Brown & Co., 1880.

15. Durack, D. T.: The weight of medical knowledge. N. Engl. J. Med. 298: 773–775, 1978.

16. Sternberg, G. M.: A contribution to the study of the bacterial organisms commonly found upon exposed mucous surfaces and in the alimentary canal of healthy individuals. Studies from the Biol. Lab. of The Johns Hopkins Univ. 2: 157–181, 1882.

17. Klebs, E.: Beiträge zur Kentnis der pathogenen Schistomyceten. VII. Die Monadinen. Arch. exp. Pathol. Pharmakol. 4: 409–488, 1875.

18. The Johns Hopkins University Register 1880–81. Baltimore: John Murphy & Co., 1881, pp 6–7.

19. Sternberg, G. M.: Experiments with disinfectants. Studies from the Biol. Lab. of the Johns Hopkins Univ. 2: 201–212, 1882.

20. Sternberg, G. M.: Induced septicaemia in the rabbit. Am. J. Med. Sci. 84: 69–76, 1882.

21. Claxton, C.: Virulence of normal human saliva. Phila. Med. Times 12: 627–631, 1882.

22. Sternberg, G. M.: Virulence of normal human saliva. Phila. Med. Times 12: 836–839, 1882.

23. Sternberg, G. M.: Virulence of normal human saliva. Phila. Med. Times 13: 80–82, 1882.

24. Neufeld, F. and Händel, L.: Weitere Untersuchungen über Pneumokokken-

Heilsera. III. Mitteilung. Über Vorkommen und Bedeutung atypiche Varietäten des Pneumokokkus. Arb. a. d. k. Gsndhtsamte. 34: 293–304, 1910.

25. Editorial: Johns Hopkins Hospital. Phila. Med. Times 13: 87, 1882.

26. Koch, R.: Zur Untersuchung von pathogenen Organismen. Mitt. a. d. k. Gshdhtsamte. 1: 1–48, 1881

27. Eberth, C. J.: Zur Kentnis der mykotischen Processe. Dtsch. Arch. f. klin. Med. 28: 1–42, 1880.

28. Friedländer, C.: Ueber die Schizomyceten bei der acuten fibrösen Pneumonie. Virchows Arch. [Pathol. Anat. u. Physiol.] 87: 319–324, 1882.

29. Friedländer, C.: Die Mikrokokken der Pneumonie. Fortschr. Med. 1: 715–733, 1883.

30. Fraenkel, A.: Ueber die genuine Pneumonie. Verhandlungen des Congress für innere Medicin. Dritter Congress 3: 17–31, 1884.

31. Günther, C.: Discussion of Leyden's report. Verhand d. Vereins f. inn. Med. z. Berlin 2: 123–125, 1882.

32. Leyden, E.: Ueber infectiöse Pneumonie. Verhand d. Vereins f. inn. Med. z. Berlin 2: 121–123, 1882.

33. Sternberg, G. M.: The Pneumonia-coccus of Friedländer (*Micrococcus Pasteuri*, Sternberg). Am. J. Med. Sci. 90: 106–123, 1885.

34. Sternberg, G. M.: The Pneumonia-coccus of Friedländer (*Micrococcus Pasteuri*, Sternberg). Second Paper. Am. J. Med. Sci. 90: 435–438, 1885.

35. Sternberg, G. M.: The etiology of croupous pneumonia. Tr. Med. Soc. State of N.Y. 53–80, 1889.

36. Sternberg, G. M.: The etiology of croupous pneumonia. Natl. Med. Rev. 7: 175–177, 1897.

37. Bergey's Manual of Determinative Bacteriology. 8th Ed. Buchanan, R. E. and Gibbons, N. E., Eds. Baltimore: Williams & Wilkins Co., pp. 499–500, 1974.

38. Report of Dr. Welch's remarks on the Diplococcus pneumoniae at the meeting of the Johns Hopkins Hospital Medical Society, on February 17th, 1890. Johns Hopkins Hosp. Bull. 1: 73–74, 1890.

39. The Johns Hopkins Hospital Medical Society Meeting of February 17th, 1890. Johns Hopkins Hosp. Bull. 1: 59, 1890.

40. Welch, W. H.: President's address. The etiology of acute lobar pneumonia considered from a bacteriological point of view. Trans. Med. Chir. Fac. State of Md., Ninety-Fourth Annual Session: 80–109, 1892.

41. Welch, W. H.: *Micrococcus lanceolatus*, with especial reference to the etiology of acute lobar pneumonia. *In* Papers and Addresses by William H. Welch, Vol II. Bacteriology. Baltimore: The Johns Hopkins University Press, pp. 146–180, 1920.

42. Osler, W.: Infectious (so-called ulcerative) endocarditis. Arch. Med. 5: 44–68, 1881.

43. Osler, W.: Gulstonian Lectures on malignant endocarditis. Lancet 1:415–418, 459–464, 505–508, 1885.

44. Osler, W.: A review of the cases studied by the third and fourth year classes, Johns Hopkins Hospital, session of 1896–1897. Natl. Med. Rev. 7: 177–180, 1897.

45. Chatard, J. A.: An analytical study of acute lobar pneumonia in the Johns Hopkins Hospital, from May 15, 1889 to May 15, 1905. Johns Hopkins Hosp. Rep.15: 55–80, 1910.

46. Emerson, C. P.: The termination of pneumonia in cases with recovery. Johns Hopkins Hosp. Rep. 15: 103–137, 1910.

47. Friedländer, C.: Weitere Bemerkungen über Pneumonie-Micrococcen. Fortschr. d. Med. 2: 333–336, 1884.

48. Futcher, T. B.: The blood in pneumonia. Natl. Med. Rev. 7: 180–182, 1897.

49. Cole, R. I.: Blood cultures in pneumonia. Johns Hopkins Hosp. Bull. 13: 136–139, 1902.

50. Cole, R. I.: Pneumococcus septicemia, meningitis and arthritis. Johns Hopkins Hosp. Bull. 13: 143–145, 1902.

51. Hanes, F.: Pneumococcus meningitis. Johns Hopkins Hosp. Rep. 15: 247–276, 1910.

52. Howard, C. P.: Pneumococcic arthritis. Johns Hopkins Hosp. Rep. 15: 229–245, 1910.

53. Herzog, H.: Beitrag zur Kenntnis der Pneumokokkenarthritis im ersten Kindersalter. Jahrb. f. Kinderh. 63: 446–469, 1906.

54. Schulz, R. Z., Warren, M. F., and Drinker, C. K.: The passage of rabbit virulent type III pneumococci from the respiratory tract of rabbits into the lymphatics and blood. J. Exp. Med. 68: 251–261, 1938.

55. Wandel, O.: Über Pneumokokkenlokalisation. Dtsch. Arch. f. klin. Med. 78: 1–38, 1903.

56. Smith, R. O. and Wood, W. B., Jr.: Cellular mechanisms of antibacterial defense in lymph nodes. I. Pathogenesis of acute bacterial lymphadenitis. J. Exp. Med. 90: 555–566, 1949.

57. Smith, R. O. and Wood, W. B., Jr.: Cellular mechanisms of antibacterial defense in lymph nodes. II. The origin and filtration effect of granulocytes in the nodal sinuses during acute bacterial lymphadenitis. J. Exp. Med. 90: 567–576, 1949.

58. Austrian, R.: The role of toxemia and of neural injury in the outcome of pneumococcal meningitis. Am. J. Med. Sci. 247: 257–262, 1964.

59. White, B.: The Biology of Pneumococcus. New York: The Commonwealth Fund, p. 227, 1938.

60. Rake, G.: Pathogenesis of pneumococcus infections in mice. J. Exp. Med. 63: 191–208, 1936.

61. Belsey, M. A.: Pneumococcal bacteremia. A report of three cases. Am. J. Dis. Child. 113: 588–589, 1967.

62. Torphy, D. E. and Ray, C. G.: Occult pneumococcal bacteremia. Am. J. Dis. Child. 119: 336–338, 1970.

63. Burke, J. P. et al.: Pneumococcal bacteremia. Review of 111 cases, 1957–1969, with special reference to cases with undetermined focus. Am. J. Dis. Child. 121: 353–359, 1971.

64. McGowan, J. E.: Bacteremia in febrile children seen in a "walk-in" pediatric clinic. N. Engl. J. Med. 288: 1309–1312, 1973.

65. Teele, D. W. et al.: Bacteremia in febrile children under 2 years of age: Results of cultures of blood of 600 consecutive febrile children seen in a "walk-in" clinic. J. Pediatr. 87: 227–230, 1975.

66. Bratton, L., Teele, D. W. and Klein, J. O.: Outcome of unsuspected pneumococcemia in children not initially admitted to the hospital. J. Pediatr. 90: 703–706, 1977.

67. Gwaltney, J. M., Jr. et al.: Spread of *Streptococcus pneumoniae* in families.

II. Relation of transfer of *S. pneumoniae* to incidence of colds and serum antibody. J. Infect. Dis. 132: 62–68, 1975.

68. Osler, W.: On certain features in the prognosis of pneumonia. Am. J. Med. Sci. 113: 1–10, 1897.

69. Thayer, W. S.: Cotton Mather's rules of health. *In* Osler and Other Papers. Baltimore: The Johns Hopkins University Press, pp. 141–164, 1931.

3

The Quellung Reaction: A Neglected Microbiologic Technique

The thing that hath been is that which shall be; and that which is done is that which shall be done: and there is nothing new under the sun.

Ecclesiastes i, 9

There are few techniques available to the diagnostic microbiologist that rival the quellung reaction for ease of performance, speed of results, accuracy, and economy. In conjunction with the Gram stain, it may permit the prompt identification of several bacterial species as components of the microbial flora of man and, when such organisms are isolated from some bodily sites, establish them as the cause of illness. These facts notwithstanding, the quellung reaction is employed with relative infrequency today. The reasons for its neglect are several, and they will be cited in the brief historical review of the technique and of its application which follows. It is hoped that these considerations may stimulate a return to the more general use of the reaction by diagnostic microbiologists.

The quellung reaction resulting from the interaction of bacterial capsular polysaccharide with homologous anticapsular antibody was discovered by Franz Neufeld and reported by him in a paper entitled: "Ueber die Agglutination der Pneumokokken und über die Theorie der Agglutination" published in 1902 in the *Zeitschrift für Hygiene und Infektionskrankheiten*.[1] He described the reaction with rabbit antiserum in the following fashion:

If one mixes equal parts of agglutinating serum and of pneumococcal broth culture, be it in a test tube or by emulsifying a loop of serum and of culture on a coverglass, one observes in the hanging drop a significantly swollen appearance which develops imme-

diately or in several minutes with a powerfully effective serum. The single cocci swell
to double and triple their size, there is flattening of their points of contact which are
otherwise tapered in relation to one another and their contours become indistinct and
blurred. Meanwhile, let it be recognized that in this quellung process, chiefly the outer
layers of the bacterial cell are concerned; they convert themselves into a homogeneous
glassy mass while in the middle of the coccus a dark round nucleus is to be seen. The
circumstance gives next the impression that, through the action of the serum, a high
grade degeneration and the beginning of the solution of the bacterium takes place. This
impression is strengthened by the fact that such swollen pneumococci have lost their
stainability. When dried and fixed in the usual fashion, they take up almost no dye; if
one adds cautiously a dye to the fluid drop, then one succeeds at most in staining the
dark kernels described in the middle of the actually swollen masses, which themselves
remain uncolored.

Application of this important observation to diagnostic microbiology was
not to take place until nearly three decades later; for, at the time it was made,
there existed few indications of the serologic heterogeneity of pneumococcus.
The reaction was cited again in 1912 by Neufeld and Händel in the second
edition of Kolle and Wasserman's *Handbuch der pathogenen Mikroorganismen*[2] and depicted in two figures for the first time. Although two years earlier,
these same workers had established clearly the existence of two discrete
serotypes of pneumococcus,[3] they apparently saw then no application of the
quellung reaction to the serotyping of the organism.

In the same year, Aoki, working in Strasbourg, described what was undoubtedly a manifestation of the quellung reaction.[4] The technique he employed to demonstrate the phenomenon differed somewhat from the conventional one, but his results are nonetheless of historic interest. Following
admixture and incubation of the sediment of a pneumococcal broth culture
with either control or homologous horse antiserum, he made air-dried preparations on slides which were stained with 1% aqueous methylene blue and
counterstained with dilute carbol fuchsin. By the application of this technique, he reached a number of interesting conclusions regarding the interaction of pneumococcus with an homologous antiserum which are hereby
quoted:[4]

1) In vitro, pneumococci form thicker and more beautiful capsules in immune serum and in immune serum containing fluids than in normal
   serum.
2) One can also observe this phenomenon in vivo. When one injects with
   living pneumococci a rabbit which has been pretreated with immune
   serum, the pneumococci surround themselves with a fine thick capsule.

3) Capsule formation proceeds more rapidly at body temperature than at lower temperature.
4) Dead pneumococci form just as fine capsules as living ones.
5) They (capsules) form in inactivated serums as well as in fresh serums.
6) The formation of the capsule is not a vital reaction but a physico-chemical one.

The foregoing observations include much of what is known about several aspects of the quellung reaction.

Considerable progress was made in the second and third decades of this century in the delineation of pneumococcal capsular types. Extending the work of Neufeld and Händel, Dochez and Gillespie defined clearly three pneumococcal types by immune reactions and assigned the remaining strains to a heterogeneous "Group IV."[5] Analogous work was carried out in South Africa by Lister, who, in 1917, identified 11 discrete serotypes.[6] By 1929, Cooper and her associates in New York had described 32 capsular types of pneumococci.[7] In all this work, the techniques used to establish the diverse types of pneumococcus had included mouse protection tests, precipitin tests, macroscopic and microscopic agglutination tests and bactericidal tests with whole blood, but not the quellung reaction.

The third edition of Kolle and Wasserman's handbook appeared in 1928 and again the chapter on pneumococcus was written by Neufeld, this time in collaboration with Schnitzer.[8] The quellung reaction is cited therein once more, together with microphotographs of the organism following exposure to homologous antiserum and to control serum. The cells were stained with dilute crystal violet. The authors seemed reluctant to recommend microscopic agglutination with homologous antiserum in a hanging drop preparation as a means of typing pneumococci, however, lest false agglutination resulting from aggregation of organisms at the drying margins of the droplet lead to misinterpretation of the results. In the same chapter, the photograph of the refractile hyaline precipitate formed by the union of type 2 pneumococcal capsular polysaccharide with homologous anticapsular rabbit serum from the paper of Schiemann and Casper[9] is reproduced. It has the same optical properties as the capsular material surrounding the pneumococcal cell following its interaction with type-specific anticapsular serum.

The first application of the quellung reaction to the identification of pneumococci was described by Neufeld and Etinger-Tulczynska in 1931 in a paper on nasal pneumococcal infection and carriage by mice, rabbits and guinea pigs.[10] Nasal swabs of inoculated animals gave rise usually to mixed bacterial cultures in their experiments. They were able, nonetheless, readily to identify pneumococci, as is indicated by the following quotation from their report:

"However, one can quickly and surely identify pneumococci if one makes use of the following fact, that they swell (quellen) markedly immediately in homologous rabbit serum (not horse serum!). One mixes on a coverglass a loop of serum bouillon culture with a loop of rabbit immune serum and observes in a hanging drop. It is very easy (also with the dry system) to recognize the markedly swollen, almost yeastlike appearing pneumococci. The absence of these forms in control droplets clinches the diagnosis." Two photographs show clearly the presence of quelled pneumococci in microscopic preparations of mixed cultures. A footnote contains the following comment: "In addition, moreover, the quellung reaction has proved simpler and more dependable for the type diagnosis of pneumococci than agglutination."

Meanwhile, the clinical application of the quellung reaction to the typing of pneumococci from patients with pneumonia was described for the first time by Armstrong in England in the same year.[11] He used an indirect method, inoculating mice intraperitoneally with sputum and examining their peritoneal exudate four hours later. Droplets of the latter were mixed with rabbit antisera to types 1, 2 or 3 or with normal rabbit serum on a glass slide, covered with a cover slip, and examined unstained. "The immediate result, in the case of a positive reaction, is a conspicuous increase in the size of the pneumococci due to conjugation of coccus and homologous antibody; Brownian movement is retarded and the pneumococci become very apparent as lanceolate bodies surrounded by a clear, highly refractive capsular zone." He was aware of Neufeld's work as indicated by the following statement: "Neufeld, twenty years ago, applied the microscopic method to typing pneumococci, but was dissatisfied with the results he obtained with Type III"; but he did not cite Neufeld in his list of references.

The following year, Armstrong[12] and Logan and Smeall,[13] in consecutive papers in the British Medical Journal, reported the application of rabbit antisera to the direct typing of pneumococci in sputum.

A major contribution to the understanding of the quellung reaction was published by Neufeld's collaborator, Etinger-Tulczynska, in 1932. Entitled "Bacterialkapseln und 'Quellungsreaktion,'"[14] the report cites the following attributes of the phenomenon: "The reaction is strongly type specific and has the following advantages over agglutination and precipitation: 1. Prompt appearance in one minute; 2. Economy in the use of immune serums; 3. Applicability also in mixed cultures; and 4. Directly in blood, organ juices, exudates and sputum." The interpretation of the reaction is stated succinctly in the following quotation: "Accordingly, the quellung reaction is identical in its essence to precipitation; only in the first case it involves carbohydrate formed in the capsule, in the second case, free (carbohydrate)."

Etinger-Tulczynska reported also the occurrence of the quellung reaction with klebsiellas (Friedländer's bacillus), streptococci and anthrax. The paper includes the following conclusion: "A *specific quellung reaction* following the addition of homologous serum will be observed only with those of the above cited bacteria which are *capsulated*. The essence of the reaction lies in the fact that the carbohydrate in the capsule precipitates and the previously invisible capsule is made visible thereby; it can also swell considerably."

Success in typing pneumococci in sputum is cited in the same report; and, in June of the following year, Neufeld and Etinger-Tulczynska published a brief paper entitled: "Rapid Diagnosis of Pneumococcal Types from the Sputum"[15] in which they described identification of the organism in sputum of 14 of 16 cases by the quellung reaction.

The publication which had probably the greatest impact on the introduction into the United States of the quellung technique for the direct typing of pneumococci in sputum was that of Sabin, which appeared in the Journal of the American Medical Association of May 15, 1933.[16] Sabin described learning the technique from Kenneth Goodner, who had visited Neufeld's laboratory at the Robert Koch Institute in Berlin and who had used the technique himself. Among the important details stressed concerning the method was the use of rabbit rather than of equine antisera in the performane of the test. Sabin studied 100 cases of pneumonia at Bellevue Hospital and identified pneumococci in 76. Among them were included 31 strains of type 1, 22 of type 2, and 4 of type 3. Types 4, 5, 7, 8 and 13 were also recognized.

Sabin's report had immediate impact. The employment of pooled antisera to 3 to 10 pneumococcal types, suggested for use in Sabin's earlier slide agglutination test[17] by Bullowa and Schuman[18] in 1930, was applied to the quellung reaction by Cooper and Walter, who reported also that pneumococci in sputum could be typed readily after two weeks' refrigeration.[19] Beckler and MacLeod described in 1935 the results of examining 760 sputum specimens for the typing of pneumococci by the Neufeld method and found it to be the most rapid and sensitive technique for this purpose in a study carefully controlled by the use of other techniques.[20]

Over the next decade, during which serum therapy of pneumococcal pneumonia was employed, albeit with declining frequency following the introduction of sulfonamides in 1938, the quellung reaction was widely used as the principal method for the identification and typing of pneumococci. In the same period, the number of recognized pneumococcal types continued to be augmented chiefly by Mørch in Denmark[21] and by Eddy[22] in the United States. Identification of pneumococci by the quellung technique was facilitated markedly by the introduction in 1963 of pneumococcal "Omni-serum," a serologic reagent containing concentrated rabbit antibodies to all 82 pneumococcal types known at that time.[23]

Despite the foregoing advances in the identification and typing of pneumococci, their application was to be short-lived. The introduction of penicillin for the treatment of pneumococcal pneumonia by Tillet and his coworkers in 1945[24] led to the abandonment of serum therapy, with its requirement for knowledge of the capsular type of the invading pneumococcus; and the importance of identifying pneumococcal types responsible for human illness became less apparent to physicians. In addition, typing serum, which had been a by-product of therapeutic serum, soon ceased to be available commercially in the United States. With the abandonment of pneumococcal typing and, concomitantly, with the discard of the technique of inoculating sputum intraperitoneally into the mouse for the isolation of pneumococci, recognition of the organism declined strikingly. As a result thereof, the view that pneumococcal pneumonia had declined significantly in frequency came to be one held rather widely by physicians in the sixth decade of this century. Reintroduction of the classic methods for the isolation and identification of pneumococci, however, has suggested, in several studies, that there has been little if any change in the attack rates of pneumococcal pneumonia in this country and abroad, whenever appropriate bacteriologic methods have been employed.

The technique of the quellung reaction is a simple one. Although several modifications are known, the following procedure has proved highly satisfactory in the writer's hands.[25] A loopful of emulsified sputum, body fluid, mouse peritoneal washings or liquid culture is spread over an area 0.5 to 1 cm in diameter on a glass slide and allowed to dry at room temperature. In similar fashion, the cells from a single colony of pneumococcus may be emulsified in a drop of sterile broth or of normal salt solution on a slide and allowed to dry. A loopful of 1% aqueous methylene blue is placed on a cover slip, and a loopful of typing serum is then applied directly to the dried spot on the slide. The residual antiserum adhering to the loop is next mixed with the methylene blue on the cover slip and then applied to and mixed with the droplet of antiserum on the slide which has been spread previously over the area of the dried preparation. The cover slip is inverted over the wet preparation and blotted lightly. A drop of immersion oil is applied to the cover slip and the preparation is examined under the oil immersion lens of a microscope with 10× ocular lenses.

For best results, it is essential to employ oblique illumination; a microscope with a fixed substage lamp will be unsuitable for this purpose. The light from an illuminator should be reflected by a substage concave mirror through the condensor so that only the left lower third of the microscopic field is brightly illuminated when viewed through a low power (10×) objective. The other factor of importance is the density of the pneumococci in the preparation. It should be limited to 50 to 100 organisms per oil immersion field. A greater number of pneumococci may result in a prozone phenomenon when homologous anticapsular serum is applied, with inhibition of the quellung reaction by the excess antigen in the preparation. This phenomenon is most likely to be encountered with pneumococci of types 3 and 37 because of the large amount of capsular polysaccharide produced by each.

Identification of individual pneumococcal types is facilitated by the combination of monospecific antisera into pools of three or more type-specific anticapsular sera. The quellung reaction is carried out with successive pools until a positive reaction is observed. The antisera to individual types comprising the pool are tested then until a type-specific reaction can be identified. Because more than one capsular type of pneumococcus may be present in a single sputum specimen (as many as five have been recognized), it is important to observe whether or not all organisms resembling pneumococci react with a given antiserum. If not, then testing with the remaining pools of antiserum should be carried out. Although uncommon, simultaneous infection of the middle ear and of the blood with two pneumococcal types has been described.

The availability of pneumococcal "Omni-serum"[23, 26] provides the physician with an invaluable reagent for the rapid identification of pneumococci. This reagent can be used not only for the recognition of pneumococci in respiratory secretions but also for the rapid diagnosis of pneumococcal meningitis, empyema, arthritis and peritonitis. The presence of pneumococci in such body fluids can be established in a matter of minutes by use of the quellung technique, and it should be employed as a routine diagnostic procedure in all hospitals for this purpose. It has become evident also that, if the diagnosis of putative pneumococcal pneumonia is to be made with a reasonable degree of accuracy, the use of the quellung reaction is required. In the current program to redevelop pneumococcal vaccines sponsored by the National Institute of Allergy and Infectious Diseases, the recognition of putative and of proved pneumococcal infection in populations under scrutiny has risen 2- to 10-fold following reintroduction of the quellung technique as a routine diagnostic procedure. Analogous results have been reported recently also from a university hospital.[27]

The quellung reaction can be utilized to facilitate the identification and typing of other bacteria pathogenic to man. The occurrence of the phenomenon with Group A (Type I) meningococci was reported in 1935 by Clapp et al.,[28] and extended later by others to organisms of Group C.[29, 30] Group B meningococci, however, fail to give a quellung reaction. Alexander used the technique for the identification of *H. influenzae* type b in 1939[31] and reported its appli-

cation to the six known capsular types of this organism in 1946.[32] Described
first by Etinger-Tulczynska,[14] the quellung reaction has become the principal
method for the typing of klebsiellas.[33] Strains of several species of streptococci may produce capsules of carbohydrate, including those of Lancefield's
Groups B[34] and F,[35] *Streptococcus salivarius*,[36] and many strains of alpha and
nonhemolytic streptococci. A number of these organisms can be recognized
by the quellung reaction.[37, 38] Although strains of Group A beta hemolytic
streptococci may produce a capsule of hyaluronic acid, this polysaccharide is
not antigenic in mammals; and the quellung reaction cannot be used to identify it.

The quellung reaction may be manifested also by bacteria of the genus
Bacillus which are endowed with capsules of polypeptide. This phenomenon
was described first by Etinger-Tulczynska[14] and elucidated by Tomcsik.[39, 40]

The interaction of a fungus with homologous rabbit antiserum to give what
may have been a quellung reaction was reported by Roger in France in 1897,[41]
five years before its description with pneuococcus by Neufeld in Germany.[1]
Roger immunized rabbits intravenously with repeated sublethal doses of live
oïdium (Candida) albicans. When the organism was inoculated into serum, it
grew poorly and in compact masses. When an aqueous suspension of cells
from such a culture stained with methylene blue was examined microscopically, its appearance was described in the following fashion: "Let us first en-
visage an isolated yeast: the protoplasm is colored as in the normal state: it has
the same appearance and dimensions. Only it is surrounded by a colorless
mass, hyaline, somewhat lightly striated, the borders of which are sinuous,
poorly delimited, of which the size is five to ten times larger than that of the
normal cuticle. The elements are rarely isolated. . . . It is easy to convince
oneself that it is not a matter of simple juxtaposition but a fusion of the cuti-
cles, of the formation of a true zooglea." The same phenomenon was observed when cells from a colony of the organism were mixed directly on a
slide with antiserum and examined microscopically. The two drawings in the
report, one of cells grown in normal serum and the other of cells grown in
immune serum, present a marked contrast, the latter resembling strikingly the
quellung reaction. Analogous reactions with other fungi have been reported in
this century, including those with *Cryptococcus neoformans* and *Sporotrichum schenckii*.[42, 43]

The nature of the quellung reaction has been the subject of considerable
study and debate as to whether or not the phenomenon involves true swelling
of the capsule.[44, 45] Regardless of how one interprets the several experimental
findings, it is clear that the combination of antibody with a capsular polymer
outside the microbial cell wall gives rise to changes in the capsule's optical
properties which are readily identifiable through the microscope. In addition,

it makes possible anatomic localization of the bacterial antigen taking part in the reaction.

The specificity of the quellung reaction is essentially no different from that of other antigen-antibody reactions; and it is possible, at times, by means thereof to identify cross reactions between different capsular types of the same species and similar reactions among organisms of different bacterial genera and species. Cross reactions among types of pneumococci are not uncommon[21, 22] and serve as a basis for the grouping of closely related serotypes in the diagnostic sera prepared by the Danish Statens Seruminstitut.[46] Many strains of alpha and nonhemolytic streptococci produce capsules which cross react with one or another of 28 different pneumococcal serotypes[38, 47] and those of *H. influenzae*,[48] klebsiellas[49] and *E. coli*[50] possessing analogous properties have been recognized as well. Although in most instances these cross reactions are unlikely to lead to confusion when the quellung reaction is employed for diagnostic purposes, they make essential employment of the Gram stain and of cultural techniques to confirm the identity of a given organism recovered in the course of an illness.

The quellung reaction requires significant levels of antibody to become manifest, and it is seldom a useful technique for the detection of specific antibodies in the serum of man. It can be employed on occasion, however, to provide confirmation of the diagnosis of bacterial endocarditis or endarteritis, when serum of the patient obtained at the time bacteremia was demonstrated gives a positive quellung reaction with the organism isolated from the blood culture.

Reaction of capsular polymers with proteins other than antibodies may give rise to optical phenomena similar to those of the quellung reaction[51] and are of interest though they play no role in diagnostic microbiology. C reactive protein, a globulin appearing in the serum of man in a variety of inflammatory states, may give rise to the quellung reaction in the presence, but not in the absence, of calcium ions with a variety of bacterial capsules composed of phosphorylated polysaccharides.[52, 53] In addition, Shin et al.[54] have used a modification of the quellung phenomenon to demonstrate the attachment of the third component of complement (C3) to a pneumococcal capsule. A positive reaction followed incubation of cells of pneumococcus type 25 in fresh guinea pig serum, washing of the cells and then treating them with specific antibody to C3.

As implied by the foregoing remarks, the quellung reaction has considerable potential utility and requires only the simplest of laboratory equipment. In conjunction with the Gram stain, it provides a rapid and reliable technique for the identification of three important human pathogens: pneumococcus, *H. influenzae* and klebsiellas, when capsulated variants of any of these species give rise to infection in man. Second, it permits identification of serotypes of several bacterial species, some of which have greater invasive powers than others of the same species. Information of this kind has utility in assessing the potential pathogenic role of an organism in a given illness when found coexisting with other organisms in secretions such as sputum, and it has also some prognostic value. Third, identification of those serotypes of a bacterial species manifesting a high degree of invasiveness and causing frequent infection plays an important role in the selection of capsular antigens for inclusion in prophylactic vaccines. Finally, serotyping of capsulated bacteria by means of the quellung reaction provides an epidemiologic tool for the identification of bacterial strains, such as those of klebsiellas, giving rise to outbreaks of nosocomial infection.[55]

Conclusion

Because of the simplicity, speed and economy of the quellung reaction, it is the writer's hope that the foregoing comments will stimulate microbiologists to make greater use of its potential than has been made in the recent past and to assure, by their concerted action, that the necessary reagents for its accomplishment will become generally available to diagnostic laboratories once again. I have known and enjoyed Stanley Schneierson for almost two decades. I think he will share my enthusiasm for the quellung reaction. Although it may be lacking in novelty, it remains a most useful and elegant bacteriologic technique.

References

1. Neufeld, F.: Ueber die Agglutination der Pneumokokken und über die Theorie der Agglutination, Zeit. f. Hyg. u. Infektionskr. 40: 54, 1902.

2. Neufeld, F. and Händel, L.: Pneumokokken. In: *Handbuch der Pathogenen Mikroorganismen*. Kolle, W. and Wasserman, A. V., eds. 2nd Ed. G. Fischer, Jena, 1912. Vol. 4, pp. 513–585.

3. Neufeld, F. and Händel, L.: Weitere Untersuchungen über Pneumokokken-Heilsera. III. Mitteilung. Über Vorkommen und Bedeutung atypischer Varietäten der Pneumokokkus, Arb. a. d. kaiser Gesundhtsamte 34: 293, 1910.

4. Aoki: Über Kapselbildung der Pneumokokken in Immunserum, Arch. f. Hyg. 75: 393, 1912.

5. Dochez, A. R. and Gillespie, L. J.: A Biologic Classification of Pneumococci by Means of Immunity Reactions, JAMA 67: 727, 1913.

6. Lister, F. S.: Prophylactic Inoculation of Man against Pneumococcal Infections and More Particularly against Lobar Pneumonia, Pub. S. Afr. Instit. Med. Res. No. 10: 308, 1917.

7. Cooper, G., Rosenstein, C., Walter, A., and Peizer, L.: The Further Separation of Types among the Pneumococci hitherto Included in Group IV and the Development of Therapeutic Antisera for these Types, J. Exp. Med. 55: 531, 1932.

8. Neufeld, F. and Schnitzer, R.: Pneumokokken. In: *Kolle, W. and Wasserman's Handbuch der pathogenen Mikroorganismen*. Kolle, W., Kraus, R. and Uhlenhuth, P., eds. 3rd Ed. G. Fischer, Jena, 1928. Vol. 4, pp. 965–970.

9. Schiemann, O. and Casper, W.: Sind die spezifisch präcipitablen Substanzen der 3 Pneumokokkentypen Haptene? Zeit. f. Hyg. u. Infektionskr. 108: 220, 1927.

10. Neufeld, F. and Etinger-Tulczynska, R.: Nasale Pneumokokken-infektionen und Pneumokokkenkeimträger im Tierversuch, Zeit. f. Hyg. u. Infektionskr. 112: 492, 1931.

11. Armstrong, R. R.: A Swift and Simple Method for Deciding Pneumococcal "Type," Brit. Med. J. 1: 214, 1931.

12. Armstrong, R. R.: Immediate Pneumococcal Typing, Brit. Med. J. 1: 187, 1932.

13. Logan, W. R. and Smeall, J. T.: A Direct Method of Typing Pneumococci, Brit. Med. J. 1: 188, 1932.

14. Etinger-Tulczynska, R.: Bakterialkapseln und "Quellungsreaction," Zeit. f. Hyg. u. Infektionskr. 114: 769, 1933.

15. Neufeld, F. and Etinger-Tulczynska, R.: Schnelldiagnose der Pneumokokken-typen aus dem Auswurf, Zeit. f. Hyg. u. Infektionskr. 115: 431, 1933.

16. Sabin, A. B.: Immediate Pneumococcus Typing Directly from Sputum by the Neufeld Reaction, JAMA 100: 1584, 1933.

17. Sabin, A. B.: The "Stained Slide" Microscopic Agglutination Test. Its Applicability to (1) Rapid Typing of Pneumococci, (2) Determination of Antibody, Am. J. Pub. Health 19: 1148, 1929.

18. Bullowa, J. G. M. and Schuman, A. H.: A Rapid Method of Using the Sabin Slide Microscopic Test for Determining the Types of Pneumococci, Am. J. Pub.Health 20: 878, 1930.

19. Cooper, G. M. and Walter, A. W.: Application of the Neufeld Reaction to the Identification of Types of Pneumococci with the Use of Antisera for Thirty-Two Types, Am. J. Pub. Health 25: 469, 1935.

20. Beckler, E. and MacLeod, P.: The Neufeld Method of Pneumococcus Type Determination as Carried Out in a Public Health Laboratory, J. Clin. Invest. 13: 901, 1934.

21. Mørch, E.: Further Studies on the Serology of the Pneumococcus Group, J. Immunol. 43: 177, 1942.

22. Eddy, B. E.: A Study of Cross Reactions among Pneumococcic Types and Their Application to the Identification of Types, Pub. Health Rep. 59: 451, 1944.

————. Cross Reactions between the Several Pneumococcic Types and Their Significance in the Preparation of Polyvalent Antiserum, ibid. 59: 485, 1944.

23. Lund, E.: Polyvalent, Diagnostic Pneumococcus Sera, Acta Path. et Microbiol. Scand. 59: 533, 1963.

24. Tillett, W. S., McCormack, J. E. and Cambier, M. J.: Treatment of Lobar Pneumonia with Penicillin, J. Clin. Invest. 24: 589, 1945.

25. Austrian, R.: *Streptococcus pneumoniae* (Pneumococcus), in Lennette, E. H., Spaulding, E. H. and Truant, J. P., eds., *Manual of Clinical Microbiology*, 2nd Ed., Am. Soc. Microbiol., Washington, D.C., 1974, pp. 109–115.

26. Lund, E. and Rasmussen, P.: Omni-Serum. A Diagnostic Pneumococcus Serum Reacting with the 82 Known Types of Pneumococcus, Acta Path. et Microbiol. Scand. 68: 458, 1966.

27. Merrill, C. W., Gwaltney, J. M., Jr., Hendley, J. O., and Sande, M. A.: Rapid Identification of Pneumococci. Gram Stain vs. the Quellung Reaction, N. Engl. J. Med. 288: 510, 1973.

28. Clapp, F. L., Phillips, S. W. and Stahl, H. J.: Quantitative Use of Neufeld Reaction with Special Reference to Titration of Type II Antipneumococcic Horse Serum, Proc. Soc. Exp. Biol. Med. 33: 302, 1935.

29. Beckler, E. A.: Meningococcus Grouping. Note on Experience with the Capsular Swelling Test, J. Lab. Clin. Med. 30: 745, 1945.

30 Milner, K. C. and Shaffer, M. A.: Type-Specific Capsular Swelling of Meningococci by Chicken Antiserum, Proc. Soc. Exp. Biol. Med. 62: 48, 1946.

31. Alexander, H. E.: Type "B" Anti-Influenza Rabbit Serum for Therapeutic Purposes, Proc. Soc. Exp. Biol. Med. 40: 313, 1939.

32. Alexander, H. E., Leidy, G. and MacPherson, C.: Production of Types A, B, C, D, E and F H. influenzae Antibody for Diagnostic and Therapeutic Purposes, J. Immunol. 54: 207, 1946.

33. Casewell, M. W.: Experiences in the Use of Commercial Antisera for the Capsular Typing of Klebsiella Species, J. Clin. Path. 25: 734, 1972.

34. Lancefield, R. C.: A Serological Differentiation of Specific Types of Bovine Hemolytic Streptococci (Group B), J. Exp. Med. 59: 441, 1934.

35. Heidelberger, M., Willers, J. M. N. and Michel, M. F.: Immunochemical Relationships of Certain Streptococcal Group and Type Polysaccharides to Pneumococcal Capsular Antigens, J. Immunol. 102: 1119, 1969.

36. Mirick, G. S., Thomas, L., Curnen, E. C. and Horsfall, F. L., Jr.: Studies on a Non-Hemolytic Streptococcus Isolated from the Respiratory Tract of Human Beings. I. Biological Characteristics of Streptococcus MG, and III. Immunological Relationships of Streptococcus MG to Streptococcus salivarius Type I, J. Exp. Med. 80: 391 and 431, 1944.

37. Willers, J. M. N., Ottens, H. and Michel, M. F.: Immunochemical Relationship between Streptococcus MG, F III and *Streptococcus salivarius*, J. Gen. Microbiol. 37: 425, 1964.

38. Austrian, R., Buettger, C. and Dole, M.: Problems in the Classification and Pathogenic Role of Alpha and Nonhemolytic Streptococci of the Human Respiratory Tract, in Wannamaker, L. W. and Matsen, J. M., eds. *Streptococci and Streptococcal Diseases*. Academic Press, New York, 1972, pp. 355–370.

39. Bodon, G. and Tomcsik, J.: Effect of Antibody on the Capsule of Anthrax Bacilli, Proc. Soc. Exp. Biol. Med. 32: 122, 1934.

40. Tomcsik, J.: Antibodies as Indicators of Bacterial Structure, Ann. Rev. Microbiol. 10: 213, 1956.

41. Roger, H.: Les Infections non bacteriennes. Recherches sur l'Oïdo-mycose, Rev. Gen. Sci. Pures et Pract. 7: 770, 1896.

42. Neill, J. M., Castillo, C. G., Smith, R. H. and Kapros, C. E.: Capsular Reactions and Soluble Antigens of Torula histolytica and of Sporotrichum schenckii, J. Exp. Med. 89: 93, 1949.

43. Evans, E. E.: Capsular Reactions of *Cryptococcus neoformans*, Ann. N.Y. Acad. Sci. 89: 184, 1960.

44. Johnson, F. H. and Dennison, W. L.: The Volume Change that Accompanies the Quellung Reaction of Pneumococci, J. Immunol. 48: 317, 1944.

45. Baker, R. F. and Loosli, C. G.: The Ultrastructure of Encapsulated *Diplococcus pneumoniae* before and after Exposure to Type Specific Antibody, Lab. Invest. 15: 716, 1966.

46. Lund, E.: Laboratory Diagnosis of *Pneumococcus* Infections, Bull. WHO 23: 5, 1960.

47. Mørch, E.: Antigenic Relationships between Pneumococcus and Non-Hemolytic Streptococci, Acta Path. et Microbiol. Scand. 27: 110, 1950.

48. Zepp, H. D. and Hodes, H. L.: Antigenic Relation of Type B *H. influenzae* to Type 29 and Type 6 Pneumococci, Proc. Soc. Exp. Biol. Med. 52: 315, 1943.

49. Heidelberger, M. and Nimmich, W.: Additional Immunochemical Relationships of Capsular Polysaccharides of Klebsiella and Pneumococci, J. Immunol. 109: 1337, 1972.

50. Robbins, J. B., Myerowitz, J. K., Whisnant, J. K., Argaman, M., Schneerson, R., Handzel, Z. T. and Gotschlich, E. C.: Enteric Bacteria Cross-Reactive with *Neisseria meningitidis* Groups A and C and *Diplococcus pneumoniae* Types I and III, Infect. and Immun. 6: 651, 1972.

51. Jacox, R. F.: A New Method for the Production of Non-Specific Capsular Swelling of the Pneumococcus, Proc. Soc. Exp. Biol. Med. 66: 635, 1947.

52. Löfstrom, G.: Comparison between the Reactions of Acute Phase Serum with Pneumococcus C- Polysaccharide and with Pneumococcus Type 27, Br. J. Exp. Path. 25: 21, 1944.

53. Bornstein, D. L., Schiffman, G., Bernheimer, H. P. and Austrian, R.: Capsulation of Pneumococcus with Soluble C-Like Polysaccharide, J. Exp. Med. 128: 1385, 1968.

54. Shin, H. S., Smith, M. R. and Wood, W. B., Jr.: Heat Labile Opsonins to Pneumococcus. II. Involvement of C3 and C5, J. Exp. Med. 130: 1229, 1969.

55. Steinhauer, B. W., Eickhoff, T. C., Kislak, J. W. and Finland, M.: The Klebsiella-Enterobacter-Serratia Division. Clinical and Epidemiologic Characteristics, Ann. Int. Med. 65: 1180, 1966.

4

Random Gleanings from a Life with the Pneumococcus

The man we honor annually with this lecture has had one of the most distinguished careers in the contemporary history of infectious diseases. Recognized throughout the world for his manifold contributions, Maxwell Finland has dealt, at one time or another, with a significant proportion of the varied problems encompassed by this area of medicine. I am privileged this evening to touch upon one of those areas to which he has made multiple contributions, that of pneumococcal infection. Pneumococcal pneumonia was a major preoccupation of Maxwell Finland during the 1920s and 1930s; and, in my own endeavors, I have had frequent occasion to draw upon his numerous publications for guidance. Although it was not my good fortune to have been one of his pupils in the restricted sense of that term, a friendship fostered by mutual interests has been most rewarding for me; and I am deeply grateful to the Infectious Diseases Society of America for this opportunity to pay tribute to one who has given so unstintingly to this organization and for whom we have such affection and admiration.

My own interest in pneumococcal infection dates from medical school days at Hopkins in the late 1930s. Sir William Osler was a keen student of pneumonia, which he termed "captain of the men of death" in the fourth edition of his famous textbook.[1] In his early years at Hopkins, he wrote: "In the rapid development of the medical curriculum, we teachers of 'bread and butter' subjects must take care that our facilities keep pace with those of the purely scientific branches. Today it is easier to train students in anatomy and physiology than in medicine and surgery. Indeed, a school may possess first-class scientific equipment with third-class clinical advantages.

"Among diseases there is not one which requires to be more fully and carefully presented than pneumonia—the most common as well as the most serious acute infection of this country, with a mortality exceeding that of all other acute fevers put together, measles, scarlet fever, diphtheria, whooping-cough, typhoid fever and dysentery."[2]

To this end, Osler established in 1896 a tradition for the third- and fourth-year medical classes of reviewing annually all of the cases of pneumonia admitted to the medical wards of the Johns Hopkins Hospital. "As our aim," he wrote, "is to make this a school of practical medicine, I dispense as far as possible with all theoretical and didactic considerations and make the cases teach the lesson of the disease."[3] The tradition endured, and I came under its influence at the time of the introduction of sulfonamides in the treatment of pneumonia. The experience was a stimulating one that had lasting impact in fostering my interests in the pneumococcus and the diseases it causes, and I have pursued these interests ever since.

Despite the advent in the past four decades of several antimicrobial drugs potent against the pneumococcus, there is little to indicate that the attack rate of pneumococcal pneumonia has changed significantly from the time prior to their availability. Evidence from several large hospitals demonstrates that as many patients with bacteremic pneumococcal pneumonia are admitted today as were admitted 40 years ago. In the country's greatly expanded population, there are still almost half as many deaths from pneumonia as there were at the turn of the century; and, although a significant number of these are the result of infections with agents other than pneumococcus, the latter still takes its toll. An analysis of deaths from bacteremic pneumococcal infection treated with bactericidal drugs suggests strongly that such deaths result from irreversible injury to the patient prior to the administration of specific antipneumococcal therapy.[4] An assessment of the contemporary magnitude of this problem and the ways of dealing with it requires consideration both of the diagnosis of pneumococcal infection and of its prophylaxis. This evening I should like to touch on certain aspects of each of these two problems, looking at both from a quasi-historical perspective, for the latter provides some interesting insights into advances in medicine.

Identification of the Pneumococcus

If one is to study pneumococcal infection, one must be able to isolate and identify the organism. Although probably first seen by Klebs[5] in 1875 in the bronchial contents of patients dying of pneumonia, pneumococcus was isolated first and almost simultaneously by Pasteur[6] and by Sternberg[7] in 1880. Pasteur, seeking the cause of rabies, recovered the organism from the blood of rabbits injected with saliva taken from the lips of a five-year-old boy who had died 4 hr earlier of this dread disease. Sternberg isolated a similar organism after injection of his own saliva into rabbits and illustrated it in his first publication. He demonstrated that the microbe was not filterable, that it was killed by heat and by carbolic acid; and he was able to grow it in a bouillon made from rabbit flesh. As illustrated by the following quotation, Sternberg clearly described the carrier state in his initial report: "Query: Does the saliva of other individuals injected in the same manner give similar results? Answer: The saliva of four students, residents of Baltimore (in March), gave negative results; eleven rabbits injected with the saliva of six individuals in Philadelphia gave eight deaths and three negative results . . ." As a former or present resident of both cities, I shall refrain from comment.

Several years were to elapse before it was established that the organism isolated by Pasteur and by Sternberg was identical with that causing lobar pneumonia. It was in that era that the acrimonious polemic between Friedländer and Fraenkel over the etiology of lobar pneumonia took place.[8] Although the organism isolated by Friedländer was the sole gram-negative bacterium found in sections from 20 of Friedländer's fatal cases of lobar pneumonia examined by Gram, neither collaborator appreciated the significance of this observation. Resolution of the issue is attributed usually to Weichselbaum, who carried out and reported an extensive study of the bacteriology of pneumonia in 1886.[9] It was he who first proposed the name *Diplococcus pneumoniae*, which was adopted by American taxonomists in 1920 for the pneumococcus.[10] In light of the fact that the official name of this organism in the United States is soon to be changed to *Streptococcus pneumoniae*, the comments in 1897 of Sternberg, co-discoverer of the pneumococcus, are of interest: "I object to the name 'diplococcus pneumoniae' because this micrococcus in certain culture media forms longer or shorter chains and it is, in fact, a streptococcus."[11] That this is so was shown indisputably by the discovery of filamentous variants of pneumococci[12, 13] and by subsequent demonstrations of the genetic relatedness of α-streptococci and pneumococci in transformation reactions.[14, 15]

In the early period of its investigation, recognition of the pneumococcus was based upon its morphology, with special emphasis on its capsule and its pathogenicity for rabbits and mice but not, in most instances, for guinea pigs. Today, in addition to its cellular and colonial morphology, we rely upon a variety of laboratory procedures to identify the pneumococcus, among them its lysis by bile or bile salts, its sensitivity to Optochin, and the Quellung reaction. It is of interest to examine the histories of these three procuedures.

The lytic effect of bile upon the pneumococcus was reported by Neufeld in 1900. One might wonder what motivated him to examine the interaction of the bacterium with so unusual a reagent. As indicated by the following quotation,[16] Neufeld knew that Koch had given a cow an injection of the bile of another bovine dead of rinderpest and rendered the former immune: "If one injects subcutaneously a healthy cow with a certain quantity of bile from an

animal dead of rinderpest, it sustains a very mild illness and is thereafter immune to this otherwise almost always fatal illness. In analogy with other im-
munizations, one might think that the bile contained either the toxin causing
rinderpest or a living attenuated modification of it." It was speculated also
that, in the initial host, some substance had developed that hindered the gen-
eralization of the infectious agent when injected along with it, giving rise to a
mild local or inapparent infection resulting in immunity.

These observations were apparently the stimulus to Neufeld to study the
action of bile on other infectious agents. With a collaborator, he "investigated
anthrax, cholera, typhus, B. coli, pyocyaneus, staphylococci, diphtheria, several strains of the haemorrhagic septicemia group, erysipelas as well as several streptococcal strains and found among them no culture that was dissolved
in a fashion similar to Fraenkel's diplococcus."[16] Neufeld followed microscopically the dissolution of the pneumococcus in broth cultures to which rabbit bile had been added, demonstrated that heat-killed pneumococci resisted
dissolution, and, by solvent extraction of bile, surmised that bile salts were
the active agents therein. His several attempts to immunize rabbits with the
bile of animals succumbing to pneumococcal septicemia, however, failed in
all but one instance. Neufeld's careful observation of pneumococcal autolysis
provoked by the detergent action of bile salts was to provide, nonetheless, a
diagnostic test of enduring usefulness and exemplifies the well-known aphorism of Pasteur that observation favors the prepared mind.

Like the preceding test, the Quellung reaction, the most accurate and simple
technique for the recognition and typing of pneumococcus, was also a discovery of Neufeld. In 1902, in a paper on the agglutination of pneumococci and
the theory of agglutination,[17] he described the reaction as follows: "If one
mixes equal parts of agglutinating serum and of pneumococcal broth culture
be it in a test tube or by emulsifying a loop of serum and of culture on a
coverglass, one observes in the hanging drop a significantly swollen appearance which develops immediately or in several minutes with a powerfully
effective serum." The discovery of the Quellung reaction, however, was an
observation ahead of its time, for little was known then of the diversity of
pneumococcal types. Although agglutination of pneumococci had been cited
by Metchnikoff[18] as early as 1891 and the serological diversity of pneumococcal types had been suggested by the studies of Besançon and Griffin in 1898,[19]
the clear delineation of pneumococcal types was not at hand when Neufeld
discovered the Quellung reaction. A quarter of a century was to elapse before
it was to be reexamined and subsequently to be applied to the diagnosis of
pneumococcal pneumonia.

Neufeld described the phenomenon again in Kolle and Wasserman's *Handbook of Pathogenic Microorganisms* in 1928[20] but seemed reluctant to recom-

mend it for general use in place of the more widely employed techniques of agglutination, precipitation, and mouse protection. Four years later, he reported with Etinger-Tulczynska[21] the usefulness of the test in detecting pneumococci in mixed cultures obtained from animals. Meanwhile, the Quellung reaction had been rediscovered in England in 1932 both by Armstrong[22] and by Logan and Smeal,[23] who recognized pneumococci in sputum by this method. It was our society's former president, Albert Sabin, who was largely responsible for introducing the Quellung reaction into the United States in 1933.[24] He described learning the technique from Kenneth Goodner at the Hospital of the Rockefeller Institute following the latter's visit to Neufeld's laboratory in Germany. Among the essential precautions to be taken in carrying out the test was the use of rabbit rather than of horse sera for typing. The method was rapidly adopted by most laboratories and over the next 15 years was employed almost universally for the identification of pneumococci as a prelude to serum therapy. Although seldom performed today, the Quellung reaction is one of the most satisfying of laboratory procedures, and, no matter how unproductive the day, I feel it hasn't been totally wasted if I have typed a pneumococcus.

The test most widely used now for the presumptive identification of pneumococcus is based on its usual sensitivity to Optochin. The history of Optochin, or ethylhydrocupreine, is an interesting one. Quinine was used early in the 20th century in the treatment of many infections. In 1911, Morgenroth and Levy, to determine whether quinine's effect on human pneumococcal infection was antibacterial or solely antipyretic, tested the drug's therapeutic efficacy in experimentally infected mice and found it lacking. Extending their studies to Optochin, a quinine derivative, they observed a protective effect.[25] These findings led to further investigations, and in 1912 Morgenroth and Kaufmann published one of the first, if not the first, report of the development of bacterial resistance to a chemotherapeutic agent in vivo.[26] Selection in vitro of pneumococcal mutants resistant to Optochin was described by Tugendreich and Russ[27] the following year, although an analogous experiment with *Bacterium coli* (now *Escherichia coli*) and malachite green had been published two years earlier.[28]

Because of the lethality of pneumococcal infection in man and the availability of only two type-specific therapeutic antisera at the time, Optochin was used experimentally in the treatment of pneumococcal pneumonia in the second decade of this century. In their extensive studies at the Rockefeller Institute, Moore and Chesney[29] confirmed in man the observations of Morgenroth and Kaufmann in mice, demonstrating a 20-fold increase in the resistance to Optochin of the pneumococcal strain isolated from a patient undergoing treatment with this drug. The combination of rapidly emerging drug resistance as well as the toxic properties of Optochin, however, led to its abandonment as a therapeutic agent.

It is a curious circumstance that so little recognition has been given to these seminal observations on the problems of drug resistance in the management of bacterial infection. No mention is made of them in the first report of pneumococcal resistance to sulfonamides in 1939,[30] and they have received scant attention since. Like Neufeld's discovery of the Quellung reaction, they were observations ahead of their time, and the interval between the discard of Optochin as a therapeutic agent and the discovery of safer and more effective antipneumococcal drugs was too long to foster their ready recollection. Mutant strains of pneumococci isolated from man and resistant to sulfonamides, tetracyclines, erythromycin, or lincomycin are now known, and, more recently, strains with increased resistance to penicillin have been identified.[31, 32] Although resistance to penicillin of pneumococcal strains from human sources has not yet reached a level sufficient to cause concern, continued monitoring of this phenomenon is warranted.

Our present familiarity with Optochin results from its recent reintroduction as a reagent for the presumptive identification of pneumococci in the general absence of typing serum. As early as 1915, Rochs in Germany[33] suggested the use of Optochin for this purpose, as did Moore in the United States.[34] This proposal was revived in 1955 by Bowers and Jeffries,[35] who employed the impregnated paper disk method. Most recently, Ragsdale and our society's Secretary, Jay Sanford, have pointed out the need to restandardize the test for cultures grown in an atmosphere of 5% CO_2.[36]

The Optochin disk method, when used in testing pure cultures, provides a presumptive identification of pneumococcus with 90%–95% accuracy. It is significantly less satisfactory, however, than the Quellung reaction, requiring more time and providing no information regarding the distribution of pneumococcal types responsible for human infection at any given time and place. It has been a source of continuing concern that there is no generally available source of high-quality diagnostic sera for the typing of pneumococci in this country; as a result, awareness of the importance of pneumococcal infection is significantly less than it should be. Contemporary students of the organism and the diseases it causes both here and abroad owe a debt of gratitude to Dr. Erna Lund[37] and the Danish State Serum Institute for continuing to make these reagents available. Together, they form a world resource upon which many are heavily dependent. The impact of capsular typing on the recognition of pneumococcus is borne out by our experiences in the pneumococcal vaccine program sponsored by the National Institute of Allergy and Infectious Diseases. Whenever routine typing of pneumococci has been reintroduced, there has been a two- to 10-fold increase in the recognition of the organism in the institution concerned. Until physicians can be reconditioned to obtain routinely cultures of blood and respiratory secretions before antimicrobial therapy and until laboratories return to optimal procedures for isolating and typing pneumococci, the true magnitude of illness caused by this organism will continue to be underestimated.

Diagnosis of Pneumococcal Infection

Not only must one be able to isolate and to identify pneumococcus, but also one must be able to demonstrate its causal role in illness, especially in pneumonia. As noted earlier, the first strains of pneumococci to be isolated in the laboratory were recovered from carriers of the organism rather than from those infected with it. The fact that the pneumococcus is part of the upper respiratory flora of a significant proportion of normal humans makes uncertain the demonstration of its causal role in disease of the lungs when it has been recovered solely from expectorated respiratory secretions. The diagnosis can be confirmed in a variety of ways: by recovery of the organism from blood or a metastatic focus of infection, by its direct isolation from the lower respiratory tract by lung or transtracheal puncture, by the detection of capsular polysaccharide in blood, urine, or other body fluids, or by the demonstration of an immunologic response to infection. Of these, the last is most likely to meet the needs of epidemiologic investigations, and it is evident that suitable methods must be available if such studies are to be undertaken.

A variety of techniques has been employed previously to this end, including agglutination, quantitative precipitation, bactericidal tests with whole blood, and mouse protection. Human antibodies to pneumococcal capsular polysaccharides do not fix complement,[38, 39] and this useful test cannot be employed, therefore, in the study of pneumococcal infection in man. Two methods developed more recently for the assay of pneumococcal antibodies include the indirect HA test of Ammann and Pelger[40] and the radioimmunoassay of Schiffman et al.[41] The latter, based upon the Farr technique,[42] and employing as antigens pneumococcal polysaccharides labeled intrinsically with ^{14}C, is the test used in the studies to be described. It has the advantages of sensitivity, being capable of detecting specific capsular antibody in the nanogram range, and of requiring very small amounts of serum for the assay procedure. In double-blind comparisons with the quantitative precipitin test, the indirect H A test, and the mouse protection test, the radioimmunoassay has given highly satisfactory results. In addition, the procedure can be modified to permit the quantification of free capsular polysaccharide and of antigen-antibody complexes in serum;[43] in its several forms, the radioimmunoassay provides a satisfactory technique for the study not only of the immunology of pneumococcal infection, but also of the antigenicity of pneumococcal vaccines.

Prophylaxis: Pneumococcal Vaccines

Having considered some aspects of the bacteriologic and immunologic diagnosis of pneumococcal infection, let us turn now to the problem of pneumonia. A study of bacteremic pneumococcal pneumonia conducted between 1952 and 1962 in New York suggests that, in the absence of more precise knowledge of the physiologic derangements that accompany pneumococcal infection and of the means to correct them, prophylaxis is the only means of reducing the mortality rate (17%) among those treated with bactericidal drugs.[4] This study showed also that those at greatest risk of a fatal outcome were individuals irreversibly injured early in the course of infection and included persons 50 years of age and older and/or ones with chronic underlying illness who were infected with one or another of a limited number of pneumococcal types.

To determine the prevalence of pneumococcal types responsible for bacteremic infection, surveillance was established in 1967 in selected city hospitals in widely separated areas throughout the nation. Since then, 3,348 such infections have been identified. In Chicago's Cook County Hospital alone, there have been 1,100 pneumococcal isolates from blood or body fluids during this period. Analysis of the types most often responsible for bacteremic infection, of which 12 account for 75%–80%, has provided the data for the selection of those to be included in vaccines in this country. It is of interest that the potential prophylactic advantage to be gained by adding successive polysaccharides to a polyvalent vaccine declines in approximately semilogarithmic fashion.

The use of pneumococcal vaccines dates from 1911, when Sir Almroth Wright investigated their potential value in preventing pneumonia among South African gold miners before the delineation of pneumococcal types.[44] In the next 40 years, both here and abroad, nearly half a million persons received polyvalent vaccines composed of either whole pneumococcal cells or their capsular polysaccharides without serious untoward reactions, but with uncertain benefit.

The discovery in 1930 of the immunogenicity of pneumococcal capsular polysaccharides in man by Francis and Tillett[45] was a fortuitous event. In the course of investigating the cutaneous reactions of patients recovering from pneumococcal pneumonia to the intradermal injection of purified capsular polysaccharides, these investigators found that antibodies developed not only to the pneumococcal type causing the infection but also to the heterologous types, the polysaccharides of which had also been injected. The potential importance of this observation was quickly recognized by Dr. Finland, who, with several collaborators, carried out a series of investigations demonstrating the antigenicity of pneumococcal polysaccharides in healthy humans and providing the first data on the relation of dosage to immunologic responsiveness.[46-52]

Subsequent investigations by Heidelberger, MacLeod, and their associates[53,54] showed that it was possible to combine six pneumococcal polysaccharides into a single vaccine, that most individuals responded to all six components of the vaccine, and that half-maximal levels of antibody persisted for five to eight years after a single injection. In our present studies, we have utilized polyvalent vaccines containing 12–14 pneumococcal capsular polysaccharides with comparable results, although none of our volunteers has been followed for longer than two years. From dose-response studies in which each of 14 capsular polysaccharides was injected in amounts ranging from 5 to 1,000 μg, a dose of 50 μg in adults has been found satisfactory whether administered as a monovalent vaccine or in polyvalent formulations.

Both monovalent and polyvalent vaccines have proved highly acceptable in terms of the low levels of untoward reactions they engender. Among several thousand recipients, approximately two-thirds have experienced no reaction whatever, and among the remainder, mild erythema and tenderness at the site of the injection have been the reactions most commonly observed. Elevation of temperature by 1°F for 12–24 hr has been noted in approximately 1% of those receiving vaccines containing 12 or more polysaccharides.

Unlike adults, infants manifest strikingly unequal responsiveness to different pneumococcal polysaccharides, although the low levels of antibody after immunization with most types are similar to those observed after injection of the capsular polysaccharides of other bacterial species.[55-57] We have assayed the sera of 30 infants given an octavalent pneumococcal vaccine by Dr. V. M. Howie of Huntsville, Ala. Although the antibody response to the type 3 capsular polysaccharide in the vaccine resembled in magnitude that seen in adults, the responses to the capsular antigens of the four pneumococcal types most often responsible for infection in this age group (types 6, 14, 19, and 23) were minimal. The biologic basis for the differences observed is presently unknown; but it is clear that, biologically, all polysaccharides are not alike. The problem merits further investigation, for pneumococcal otitis media persists as one of the most common contemporary infections of infancy and early childhood, with an attack rate estimated to be between 15 and 20 per 100 in the first two years of life.

The safety and antigenicity of the polyvalent vaccines of pneumococcal capsular polysaccharides having been demonstrated in adults, it remained to establish the efficacy of the vaccines in preventing pneumococcal pneumonia. The first large-scale trials of a polysaccharide vaccine were carried out in the 1930s by Eckwurzel and his associates.[58] They immunized more than 61,000 adult males with a vaccine containing 1 mg each of the capsular polysaccharides of pneumococcal types 1 and 2; the study included an equal number of matched controls. Although the results of these trials were viewed as inconclusive by their initiators, they were strongly suggestive of the efficacy of the vaccine in reducing disease caused by pneumococcal types 1 and 2.

With a vaccine containing four capsular polysaccharides, MacLeod et al.[59] provided convincing evidence of its efficacy during a military epidemic of pneumococcal pneumonia in World War II. They were able to demonstrate, in a controlled study involving 17,000 young adult males, that injection of 50 μg each of the capsular polysaccharides of pneumococcal types 1, 2, 5, and 7 afforded complete protection against infection with these types in the period beginning two weeks after immunization. The two-week interval was required to develop protective levels of antibody. At approximately the same time, Kaufman provided data indicating the value of a trivalent vaccine in preventing pneumonia caused by types 1, 2, and 3 in persons of both sexes over the age of 50.[60] As a result of these studies, two hexavalent pneumococcal vaccines of different composition were developed after the war. Although licensed, they became available at a time when interest in pneumococcal infection was at its nadir, and because of their failure to be used, both were withdrawn from the market, and the license to produce them was revoked without prejudice.

To obtain licensure of the newly developed pneumococcal vaccines containing 12 or more capsular polysaccharides, several trials similar to those cited have been initiated to demonstrate their efficacy. In the present climate of research involving human subjects, it seems relevant to note that the protocol of each trial, both in this country and abroad, has been subject to multiple reviews and approval before its initiation and that appropriate informed consent is obtained before the entry of each participant into the trials.

The first study of the efficacy of these vaccines was designed to assess their impact in preventing pneumococcal pneumonia among inpatients at the Dorothea Dix Hospital, Raleigh, N.C., in collaboration with Mr. B. Mora and Dr.

W. J. Buffaloe. Because of the relatively small size of the population at risk, the results of this trial have not yet achieved statistical significance, although current trends point to the efficacy of the vaccine.

Significant results have been developed from a trial conducted in Africa. Pneumococcal pneumonia has been epidemic in African mining populations for more than 50 years and stimulated the first efforts to prevent it by vaccination.[44] The epidemiologic pattern of the infection suggests that it is unrelated to the occupation of mining per se but is similar to so-called "recruit disease," which occurs when young adults from widely dispersed geographic areas are congregated in barracks. Among populations of miners, in which both pneumococcal pneumonia and meningococcal meningitis are epidemic, the preponderance of illness occurs in the first six months of employment. The attack rate of putative pneumococcal pneumonia reaches levels exceeding 200 per 1,000 per annum. In one such population of 17,000 men with an annual turnover of 5,000, a trial with a hexavalent pneumococcal vaccine was initiated in August 1972. From a table of random numbers, men were assigned to one of three groups to receive a vaccine containing 50 μg each of the capsular polysaccharides of pneumococcal types 1, 3, 4, 7, 8, and 12, a vaccine containing 50 μg of the capsular polysaccharide of group A *Neisseria meningitidis*, or a saline placebo. In all, 4,497 men were enrolled in the trial; vaccinations were completed in June 1973. Because the term of employment for most participants is 18 months, the trial will end in January 1975.

The results of the trial were last assessed in March 1974. At that time, there had been 14 cases of radiologically confirmed pneumonia associated with the types in the vaccine among the pneumococcal vaccinees and 132 such illnesses in subjects in the two control groups. Although serologic assays are incomplete, it is evident, on the basis of clinical, radiologic, and bacteriologic criteria, that there has been an 80% reduction among vaccinees in the incidence of pneumonia associated with those pneumococcal types in the pneumococcal vaccine; the observed differences from the two control groups have a P value of <0.0001 by the χ^2 test. In addition, the efficacy of three individual components of the vaccine (types 1, 8, and 12) has been demonstrated.

More convincing evidence of the effectiveness of the vaccine is available from an analysis of its impact on bacteremic infection in which the causal infectious role of pneumococcus is unequivocally established. Among 44 such infections caused by types in the vaccine, two (both attributable to pneumococcus type 1) have occurred in pneumococcal vaccinees and the remaining 42 in the control populations. Again, the difference is highly significant (P <0.0001), and the efficacy of the vaccine in preventing or reducing the incidence of bacteremic infection with types 1 and 12 is also demonstrable. In this initial African trial, two epidemic pneumococcal types were excluded purposely from the vaccine to serve as internal controls. Analysis of bacteremic infection caused by these and other excluded pneumococcal types shows that protection stimulated by the capsular antigens is type-specific.

Because a vaccine of six capsular polysaccharides protects against too narrow a spectrum of pneumococcal infection both here and abroad, vaccines containing 12–14 capsular polysaccharides have been prepared and are currently under investigation. A second African trial, similar in structure to the one cited earlier, began in January 1974; 2,600 men have been enrolled to date, a third of whom have received a tridecavalent pneumococcal vaccine. This trial will continue for 18 months to two years.

More recently, in San Francisco, a study designed to assess the efficacy of a dodecavalent pneumococcal vaccine containing the capsular polysaccharides of pneumococcal types 1, 3, 4, 6, 7, 8, 9, 12, 14, 18, 19, and 23 has been initiated at the Kaiser Permanente Medical Center under the direction of Dr. Marvin A. Freid. Approximately 12,000 members of the Health Plan 45 years of age and older, half of whom received the vaccine, have enrolled in this investigation. The results of this trial will also be available two years hence.

What should be the anticipated impact of polyvalent vaccines of pneumococcal polysaccharides, and to whom should they be given? As noted by Heffron in 1939,[61] when lobar pneumonia was still a major concern, the true incidence of pneumococcal infection of the lungs had never been determined in this country. Now that pneumococcal pneumonia is no longer a reportable disease and with the abandonment of pneumococcal typing by most hospital laboratories, our information is still more fragmentary. On the basis of studies conducted collaboratively with Dr. Freid in San Francisco in persons 18 years of age and older, and with use of more stringent criteria for diagnosis, including immunologic confirmation thereof, one arrives at a minimal incidence of pneumococcal pneumonia in adults of two per 1,000 per annum, or approximately 420,000 such illnesses annually in the United States at the present time. If one makes the assumptions (1) that 70% of the infections are caused by types in the dodecavalent vaccine, (2) that the vaccine is 80% effective, (3) that 25% of infections are bacteremic, with an overall fatality rate of 17%, then there should be a potential saving of 17,000 lives annually in this country if the vaccine were widely employed. In contrast to the ages at which the mortality rate is highest, the peak incidence of hospital admissions for bacteremic pneumococcal pneumonia is during the fourth and fifth decades of life; and, although the mortality rate at these ages is lower, the economic burden resulting from lost productivity is significantly greater than that resulting from illness in the elderly.

Several segments of the population at greater than average risk of fatal pneumococcal infection can be identified. They include persons 50 years of age and older in whom a trivalent pneumococcal vaccine has been shown previously to be effective,[60] persons with a variety of chronic systemic illnesses, persons with a sickle cell disease,[62] and splenectomized individuals.[63, 64] Although the increased risk of pneumococcal infections in those with sicklemia is greatest in infancy, when the serologic response to several pneumococcal antigens is minimal, it persists into later life, when such individuals have been shown to develop antibodies to pneumococcal capsular polysaccharides after immunization. The potential usefulness of pneumococcal vaccines in the prevention of otitis media remains to be assessed. The extraordinary frequency of this illness of infancy and early childhood and the lasting auditory disability it causes in socioeconomically deprived populations make this area of investigation one of paramount importance for the near future.

Problems for Future Research

I have had a good time with the pneumococcus over a period of more than three decades. Although thrust aside to some extent as a result of the extraordinary therapeutic advances in the past quarter of a century, it has been the source of some of the most fundamental advances in biology and in our understanding of infectious disease in the nearly 100 years since its discovery. Despite these achievements, a number of problems worthy of study remain, some of which may be solved by persons who are in this room this evening. Among them, I would include the following: (1) Why are some pneumococcal types more invasive than others, not only in man but also in other animal species? (2) Why are certain pneumococcal types more prone to cause infection in infancy than in adult life? (3) Why do infants respond poorly to vaccines of some bacterial polysaccharides and well to others? (4) Why do some adults show an immunologic response to most pneumococcal capsular antigens but not to others? (5) Why do the anticapsular antibodies of man and of other species that produce them after immunization with pneumococcal capsular polysaccharides fail to fix complement, in contrast to the formation of complement-fixing antibodies by species that require the whole organism for immunization? (6) What is the biologic function of C-reactive protein, the abnormal globulin that appears in the circulation in a variety of inflammatory states and precipitates the cell wall polysaccharide of the pneumococcus in the presence of calcium ions? (7) Finally, and perhaps most important, how does the pneumococcus injure the mammalian host it invades?

Until we know the answer to the last of these questions, it is unlikely that we shall be able to improve further the outlook of those stricken with pneumococcal infection. Osler was well aware that the toxemia of infection was responsible for the lethality of pneumococcal pneumonia:[65] "The toxemia is the important element in the disorder to which in the majority of cases the degree of pyrexia and the consolidation are entirely subsidiary. The poisonous factors may develop early and cause from the outset severe cerebral symptoms and they are not necessarily proportionate to the degree of lung involved. There may be severe and fatal toxemia with consolidation of only one-half a lobe, while the patient with complete solidification of one lobe or of a whole lung may from beginning to close of the attack have no delirium . . .

"Very large areas of the breathing surface may be cut off without disturbing the cardiorespiratory mechanism. In no way is this more strikingly shown than by the condition of the patient after the crisis. On one day with a lung consolidated from apex to base, the respirations from 60 to 65 and the temperature between 104° and 105°, the patient may seem in truly desperate condition, and it would appear rational to attribute the urgent dyspnoea and the slight cyanosis to the mechanical interference with the exchange of gases in the lungs. But on the following day, dyspnoea and cyanosis may have disappeared, the temperature is normal and the pulse-rate greatly lessened, and yet the physical condition of the lungs remains unchanged. We witness no more striking phenomenon than this in the whole range of clinical work and its lesson is of prime importance in this very question, showing that the fever and the toxins rather than the solid exudate are the essential agents in causing cardio-respiratory symptoms . . .

"The toxemia outweighs all other elements in the prognosis of pneumonia; to it (the gradual failure of strength or more rarely in a sudden death, as here given) is due in great part the terrible mortality from this common disease and unhappily against it we have as yet no reliable measures at our disposal."

What Osler wrote of pneumonia in 1897 remains largely true today. Here is a problem worthy of the attention of our best minds and our most imaginative investigators. Until it is solved, there may be a place for pneumococcal vaccines in our prophylactic armamentarium.

In closing, I should like to express once again my appreciation to the Infectious Diseases Society of America for this opportunity to pay tribute to Dr. Finland; he has been and will continue to be, for many years to come, an inspiration to all who would till the vineyards of the medical sciences.

References

1. Osler, W. The principles and practice of medicine. 4th ed. D. Appleton, New York, 1901, p. 108.

2. Osler, W. On the study of pneumonia. St. Paul Med. J. 1: 5–9, 1899.

3. Osler, W. Pneumonia. A review of the cases studied by the third and fourth year classes, Johns Hopkins Hospital, session of 1896–97. Natl. Med. Rev. 7: 177–180, 1897.

4. Austrian, R., Gold, J. Pneumococcal bacteremia with especial reference to bacteremic pneumococcal pneumonia. Ann. Intern. Med. 60: 759–776, 1964.

5. Klebs, E. Beiträge zur Kentnis der pathogenen Schistomyceten. VII. Die Monadinen. Arch. exp. Pathol. 4: 409–488, 1875.

6. Pasteur, L. [with M M. Chamberland and Roux]. Sur une maladie nouvelle, provoquée par la salive d'un enfant mort de la rage. C. r. Acad. Sci. [D] (Paris) 92: 159–165, 1881.

7. Sternberg, G. M. A fatal form of septicemia in the rabbit, produced by subcutaneous injection of human saliva. Natl. Board of Health Bull. 2: 781–783, 1881.

8. Austrian, R. The gram stain and the etiology of lobar pneumonia, an historical note. Bacteriol. Rev. 24: 261–265, 1960.

9. Weichselbaum, A. Ueber die Aetiologie der acuten Lungen- und Rippenfellentzündungen. Med. Jahrbücher. 1: 483–554, 1886.

10. Winslow, C.-E. A., Broadhurst, J., Buchanan, R. E., Krumwiede, C., Jr., Rogers, L. A., Smith, G. H. The families and genera of the bacteria. Final report of the committee of the Society of American Bacteriologists on characterization and classification of bacterial types. J. Bacteriol. 5: 191–229, 1920.

11. Sternberg, G. M. The etiology of croupous pneumonia. Natl. Med. Rev. 7: 175–177, 1897.

12. Dawson, M. H. Variation in the pneumococcus. J. Pathol. Bacteriol. 39: 323–344, 1934.

13. Austrian, R. Morphologic variation in pneumococcus. I. An analysis of the bases for morphologic variation in pneumococcus and description of a hitherto undefined morphologic variant. J. Exp. Med. 98: 21–34, 1953.

14. Bracco, R. M., Krauss, M. R., Roe, A. S., MacLeod, C. M. Transformation reactions between pneumococcus and three strains of streptococci. J. Exp. Med. 106: 247–259, 1957.

15. Austrian, R., Buettger, C., Dole, M. Problems in the classification and pathogenic role of alpha and nonhemolytic streptococci of the human respiratory tract. *In* L. W. Wannamaker and J. M. Matson [ed.]. Streptococci and streptococcal diseases. Academic Press, New York, 1972, p. 355–370.

16. Neufeld, F. Ueber ein specifische bacteriolytische Wirkung der Galle. Z. Hyg. Infektionskr. 34: 454–464, 1900.

17. Neufeld, F. Ueber die Agglutination der Pneumokokken und über die Theorieen der Agglutination. Z. Hyg. Infektionskr. 40: 54–72, 1902.

18. Metchnikoff, E. Études sur l'immunité. IV. L'Immunité des cobayes vaccinées contre le Vibrio Metchnikowii. Ann. Inst. Pasteur 5: 465–478, 1891.

19. Bezançon, F., Griffin, V. Pouvoir agglutinatif du sérum dans les infections expérimentales et humaines à pneumocoques. C. r. Soc. Biol. 48: 579–581, 1897.

20. Neufeld, F., Schnitzer, R. Pneumokokken. *In* W. Kolle, R. Krauss, and P. Uhlen-

huth [ed.]. Handbuch der pathogenen Mikroorganismen. Vol. 4. 3rd ed. G. Fischer, Jena, 1928, p. 965–970.

21. Neufeld, F., Etinger-Tulczynska, R. Nasale Pneumokokkeninfektionen und Pneumokokkenkeimträger im Tierversuch. Z. Hyg. Infektionskr. 112: 492–526, 1931.

22. Armstrong, R. R. Immediate pneumococcal typing. Br. Med. J. 1: 187–188, 1932.

23. Logan, W. R., Smeall, J. T. A direct method of typing pneumococci. Br. Med. J. 1: 188–189, 1932.

24. Sabin, A. B. Immediate pneumococcus typing directly from sputum by the Neufeld reaction. J.A.M.A. 100: 1584–1586, 1933.

25. Morgenroth, J., Levy, R. Chemotherapie der Pneumokokkeninfektion. Klin. Wochenschr. 48: 1560–1561, 1979–1983, 1911.

26. Morgenroth, J., Kaufmann, M. Arzneifestigkeit bei Bakterien (Pneumokokken). Z. Immunitätsforsch. [I] 15: 610–624, 1912.

27. Tugendreich, J., Russo, C. Ueber die Wirkung von Chinaalkaloiden auf Pneumokokkenkulturen. Z. Immunitätsforsch. [I] 19: 156–171, 1913.

28. Seiffert, G. Studien zur Biologie der Darmbakterien. I. Fütterungsversuche mit körperfremden Kolistämmen. Dtsch. med. Wochenschr. 37: 1064–1067, 1911.

29. Moore, H. F., Chesney, A. M. A study of ethylhydrocuprein (Optochin) in the treatment of acute lobar pneumonia. Arch. Intern. Med. 19: 611–682, 1917.

30. MacLean, I. H., Rogers, K. B., Fleming, A. M. & B. 693 and pneumococci. Lancet 1: 562–568, 1939.

31. Hansman, D., Glasgow, H., Sturt, J., Devitt, L., Douglas, R. Increased resistance to penicillin of pneumococci isolated from man. N. Engl. J. Med. 284: 175–177, 1971.

32. Tempest, B., Carney, J. P., Eberle, B. Distribution of the sensitivities to penicillin of types of Diplococcus pneumoniae in an American Indian population. J. Infect. Dis. 130: 67–69, 1974.

33. Rochs, K. Zur Differentialdiagnose der Streptokokken und Pneumokokken. Virchows Arch. 220: 327–346, 1915.

34. Moore, H. F. The action of ethylhydrocuprein (Optochin) on type strains of pneumococci in vitro and in vivo, and on some other microorganisms in vitro. J. Exp. Med. 22: 269–285, 1915.

35. Bowers, E. F., Jeffries, L. R. Optochin in the identification of Str. pneumoniae. J. Clin. Pathol. 8: 58–60, 1955.

36. Ragsdale, A. R., Sanford, J. P. Interfering effect of incubation in carbon dioxide on the identification of pneumococci by Optochin discs. Appl. Microbiol. 22: 854–855, 1971.

37. Lund, E. Polyvalent, diagnostic pneumococcus sera. Acta Pathol. Microbiol. Scand. 59: 533–536, 1963.

38. Horsfall, F. J., Jr., Goodner, K. Lipids and immunological reactions. II. Further experiments on the relation of lipids to the type-specific reactions of antipneumococcus sera. J. Immunol. 31: 135–140, 1936.

39. Stats, D., Bullowa, J. G. M. Failure of the human convalescent type-specific anti-pneumococcic antibody to fix complement. J. Immunol. 44: 41–47, 1942.

40. Ammann, A. J., Pelger, R. J. Determination of antibody to pneumococcal polysaccharides with chromic chloride-treated human red blood cells and indirect hemagglutination. Appl. Microbiol. 24: 679–683, 1972.

41. Schiffman, G., Austrian, R. A radioimmunoassay for the measurement of pneumococcal capsular antigens and of antibodies thereto. Fed. Proc. 30: 658, 1971.

42. Farr, R. S. A quantitative immunochemical measure of the primary interaction of I*BSA and antibody. J. Infect. Dis. 103: 239–262, 1958.

43. Schiffman, G., Summerville, J. E., Castagna, R., Douglas, R., Bonner, M. J., Austrian, R. Quantitation of antibody, antigen, and antigen-antibody complexes in sera of patients with pneumococcal pneumonia. Fed. Proc. 33: 758, 1974.

44. Wright, A. E., Parry Morgan, W., Colebrook, L., Dodgson, R. W. Observations on prophylactic inoculation against pneumococcus infections, and on the results which have been achieved by it. Lancet 1: 1–10, 87–95, 1914.

45. Francis, T., Jr., Tillett, W. S. Cutaneous reactions in pneumonia. The development of antibodies following the intradermal injection of type-specific polysaccharide. J. Exp. Med. 52: 573–585, 1930.

46. Sutliff, W. D., Finland, M., Jackson, H., Jr. Natural immunity of man to the pneumococcus. J. Clin. Invest. 10: 660–661, 1931.

47. Finland, M., Sutliff, W. D. Specific cutaneous reactions and circulating antibodies in the course of lobar pneumonia. I. Cases receiving no serum therapy. J. Exp. Med. 54: 637–652, 1931.

48. Finland, M., Sutliff, W. D. Specific antibody response of human subjects to intracutaneous injection of pneumococcus products. J. Exp. Med. 55: 853–865, 1932.

49. Finland, M., Dowling, H. F. Cutaneous reactions and antibody response to intracutaneous injections of pneumococcus polysaccharides. J. Immunol. 29: 285–299, 1935.

50. Finland, M., Ruegsegger, J. M. Immunization of human subjects with the specific carbohydrates of Type III and the related Type VIII pneumococcus. J. Clin. Invest. 14: 829–832, 1935.

51. Ruegsegger, J. M., Finland, M. The influence of dosage and route of injection on the antibody response of human subjects to the specific carbohydrate of the Type VIII pneumococcus. J. Clin. Invest. 14: 833–836, 1935.

52. Finland, M., Brown, J. W. Reactions of human subjects to the injection of purified type specific pneumococcus polysaccharides. J. Clin. Invest. 17: 479–488, 1938.

53. Heidelberger, M., MacLeod, C. M., diLapi, M. M. The human antibody response to simultaneous injection of six specific polysaccharides of pneumococcus. J. Exp. Med. 88: 369–372, 1948.

54. Heidelberger, M., deLapi, M. M., Siegel, M., Walter, A. W. Persistence of antibodies in human subjects injected with pneumococcal polysaccharides. J. Immunol. 65: 535–541, 1950.

55. Goldschneider, I., Lepow, M. L., Gotschlich, E. C., Mauck, F. T., Bachl, F., Randolph, M. Immunogenicity of group A and group C meningococcal polysaccharides in human infants. J. Infect. Dis. 128: 769–776, 1973.

56. Monto, A. S., Brandt, B. L., Artenstein, M. S. Response of children to *Neisseria meningitidis* polysaccharide vaccines. J. Infect. Dis. 127: 394–400, 1973.

57. Smith, D. H., Peter, G., Ingram, D. L., Harding, A. L., Anderson, P. Response of children immunized with the capsular polysaccharide of *Hemophilus influenzae*, type b. Pediatrics 52: 637–644, 1973.

58. Ekwurzel, G. M., Simmons, J. S., Dublin, L. I., Felton, L. D. Studies on immunizing substances in pneumococci. VIII. Report on field tests to determine the prophylactic value of a pneumococcus antigen. Public Health Rep. 53: 1877–1893, 1938.

59. MacLeod, C. M., Hodges, R. G., Heidelberger, M., Bernhard, W. G. Prevention of pneumococcal pneumonia by immunization with specific capsular polysaccharides. J. Exp. Med. 82: 445–465, 1945.

60. Kaufman, P. Pneumonia in old age. Arch. Intern. Med. 79: 518–531, 1947.

61. Heffron, R. Pneumonia with special reference to pneumococcus lobar pneumonia. Commonwealth Fund, New York, 1939, pp. 258–260.

62. Barrett-Connor, E. Bacterial infection and sickle cell anemia. An analysis of 250 infections in 166 patients and a review of the literature. Medicine (Balt.) 50: 97–112, 1971.

63. Bisno, A. L., Freeman, J. C. The syndrome of asplenia, pneumococcal sepsis, and disseminated intravascular coagulation. Ann. Intern. Med. 72: 389–393, 1970.

64. Eraklis, A. J., Kevy, S. V., Diamond, L. K., Gross, R. E. Hazard of overwhelming infection after splenectomy in childhood. N. Engl. J. Med. 276: 1225–1229, 1967.

65. Osler, W. On certain features in the prognosis of pneumonia. Am. J. Med. Sci. 113: 1–10, 1897.

5

Pneumococcus: The First One Hundred Years

In the introduction to his brilliant monograph *The Biology of Pneumococcus*, published in 1938,[1] Benjamin White wrote the following paragraphs:

Pneumococcus is an altogether amazing cell. Tiny in size, simple in structure, frail in make-up, it possesses physiological functions of great variety, performs feats of extraordinary intricacy and, attacking man, sets up a stormy disease so often fatal that it must be reckoned as one of the foremost causes of human death. Furthermore, living or dead, whole or in part, on entering the animal body, Pneumococcus starts a train of impulses, stimulating all reactions grouped under those inclusive phenomena known as immunity.

The study of the membrane of this small group of microoganisms in a subordinate branch of biology is bringing light into some of the obscure realms of the related sciences. The peculiarities of Pneumococcus are yielding a generous return to the investors and speculators who have cast in their resources with its lot, resulting in the accumulation of a store of solid bullion for the scientist and for mankind.

This year marks the centennial of the first isolations of that remarkable organism known as *Streptococcus pneumoniae*, an occasion that has motivated the holding of this conference. It will be my purpose to review briefly some of the landmarks in the history of our knowledge of the pneumococcus in the hope that this review will highlight how much can be learned from the study of a single bacterium even though the road may have been, at times, not altogether a smooth one.

Although probably visualized in pulmonary tissues by Klebs[2] as early as 1875 and by Koch[3] and Eberth[4] prior to its recovery in the laboratory, the pneumococcus was first isolated by Sternberg[5] in the United States and by Pasteur[6] in France in the second half of 1880. Sternberg, who spent almost his entire career as a member of the Medical Department of the U.S. Army and was the founder of the Army Medical School, was working in New Orleans on the etiology of malarial fever in the autumn of that year. As a control in one of his experiments, he injected his saliva subcutaneously into a rabbit. His initial findings, reported orally to the Medical and Chirurgical Faculty of Maryland and published shortly thereafter, were described by him in April 1881, in the following manner:

In a report (not yet published) made to the National Board of Health in February last, I have given a detailed account of certain experiments, made in the first instance as a check upon experiments relating to the so-called *Bacillus malariae* of Klebs and Tommasi-Crudeli, which show that my own saliva has remarkably virulent properties when injected into the subcutaneous tissue of a rabbit. Further experiments, made in the biological laboratory of the Johns Hopkins University, have fully confirmed the results heretofore obtained, and the object of the present report is to place upon the record these last experiments which are of special interest just now because of the announcement by Pasteur of "*a new disease*" produced in rabbits by the subcutaneous injection of the saliva of an infant which died of hydrophobia in one of the hospitals of Paris (Comptes Rendus Ac. d. sc. 1881, xcii, p 159).

I have demonstrated by repeated experiments that my saliva in doses of $1.25c^3$ to $1.75c^3$ (see note 1) injected into the subcutaneous connective tissue of a rabbit, infallibly produces death within forty-eight hours.

In the same report, Sternberg described the presence, in the blood of infected rabbits, of an "immense number of micrococci, usually joined in pairs and having a diameter of 0.5μ."

Pasteur's initial isolation of the pneumococcus was made in December 1880 but was reported three months before Sternberg's initial publication; this sequence gave the priority of discovery to Pasteur despite the fact that his recovery of the organism postdated that of Sternberg. In his early description of the organism, Pasteur made note of what is now recognized as the pneumococcal capsule: "Each of these little particles is surrounded at a certain focus with a sort of aureole which corresponds perhaps to a material substance."

It is noteworthy that both of the two initial isolates of the pneumococcus were obtained from carriers of the organism rather than from individuals ill with pneumococcal disease. The association of the pneumococcus with pneumonia and with infection of other bodily sites, however, was not to be long delayed, although its causal role in the former illness was to be the subject of a bitter polemic between Carl Friedländer and Albert Fraenkel. Friedländer's first report on the bacteriology of pneumonia appeared in 1882 in a communication describing the organisms found in sections of the lungs of eight patients who died from that disease.[7] It is altogether probable that he was looking at the pneumococcus. The following year he reported the isolation of the organism that now bears his name (and has the species name *Klebsiella pneumoniae*) from the right upper lobe of a patient with pneumonia and cirrhosis of the liver.[8] He recovered, from two additional cases of pneumonia, organisms that were probably pneumococci. This report contains also the first published reference to the stain of Gram, who was working in Friedländer's laboratory on a stain to facilitate the recognition of bacteria in histologic preparations. In 1884 Fraenkel described the isolation of an organism from a fatal case of pneumonia; this organism differed from Friedländer's initial isolate in its growth characteristics, and Fraenkel took exception to Friedländer's conclusions.[9] The relative roles of Friedländer's bacillus and of the pneumococcus as causes of pneumonia were to be defined by Weichselbaum[10] in 1886. These roles could have been clarified much earlier as is indicated in the following passage from Gram's original report of the stain that bears his name and that appeared in 1884.[11] In stained sections of the lungs of 20 fatal cases of pneumonia, the organisms in 19 failed, like pneumococci, to be decolorized; i.e., they were gram-positive. Of the 20th case, Gram wrote as follows: "One case of croupous pneumonia with capsulecoccus. Here one finds very many cocci which do not all lie in the cells of the exudate. They decolorize very easily in alcohol and, what is more, with and without treatment with iodine. From this case stem a great part of the cultures of Friedländer." Had either Friedländer or Gram appreciated the significance of this observation, the polemic with Fraenkel as to the principal cause of pneumonia might have been avoided and the role of pneumococcus established several years earlier.[12]

In the same decade, investigators in other countries, as well as those in Germany, contributed significantly to the understanding of pneumococcal disease. Pneumococci were recovered directly from the lung during life by Günther[13] and by Leyden[14] in 1882 and from blood obtained from the finger of a moribund patient by Talamon[15] in 1883. Friedländer[16] was also probably successful in demonstrating bacteremia by successful culture of an incompletely identified organism from one of six patients, the material for study having been obtained by cupping. Osler[17] saw what probably were pneumococci on heart valves in 1881, and, before the end of the decade, Netter[18] had produced experimental pneumococcal endocarditis in the rabbit. He also conducted studies of pneumococcal meningitis.[19] Infection of the middle ear of an adult by pneumococcus was reported by Zaufel[20] in Prague in 1887, and pneumococcal arthritis was identified two years later.[21] In the 10-year period following the initial isolation of pneumococcus, therefore, the range of pneumococcal infection had been elucidated with remarkable speed. Sternberg's interest in the pneumococcus continued for more than a decade. In his final paper on the subject,[22] he wrote, "I object to the same 'diplococcus pneumoniae' because this micrococcus in certain culture media forms longer or shorter chains and it is, in fact, a streptococcus." He would have been pleased, I think, by the belated recognition of this fact by American microbiologists.

The defenses of the host against pneumococcal infection were a subject of concern to early investigators of this disease. At the time, antitoxic and lytic activities of antisera were being recognized, but the potential role of leukocytes in host defenses was poorly understood. That recovery from infection rendered the experimental animal immune was probably suggested first by Fraenkel,[23] who challenged a rabbit after its recovery from an infection of the ear that remained localized, perhaps because of the lower temperature of the ear. The protective effect of antiserum was demonstrated in 1891 by the Klemperers,[24] who also worked with rabbits and showed that the offspring of immunized animals were resistant to challenge with the homologous strain of pneumococcus. These observations led to the first injections of immune serum into patients by the Klemperers. The rational use of serotherapy, however, had to await the recognition of the diversity of pneumococcal capsular types, which did not begin to emerge clearly until 1910.[25]

The importance of leukocytes in the defense against pneumococcal infection was suggested first by Gamaléia,[26] who worked at the Pasteur Institute. In 1888 he wrote:

We believe to have proved in this memoir

That the *streptococcus lanceolatus* of Pasteur is always found in the fibrinous pneumonia of man and that this can be revealed experimentally;

That this streptococcus produces in partially refractory animals a fibrinous inflammation of the lungs;

That its pathogenic influence is held in check in healthy human beings by the activity of the pulmonary phagocytes; . . .

Gamaléia chose the mouse for many of his experiments because it was much more susceptible to pneumococcus than was the rabbit. The mouse was so susceptible, in fact, that he suggested in a charming footnote that it might play a role as a vector in the transmission of pneumonia to humans. He was forced to abandon this hypothesis after his failure to infect mice by feeding them infected spleens. It was Issaeff,[27] a pupil of Metchnikoff, who showed that immune serum lacked both antitoxic and antibacterial properties but did promote phagocytosis. It remained for Neufeld and Rimpau[28] to demonstrate in 1904, however, that the effect of the immune serum was on the pneumococcus and not on the white cell. They showed that white cells treated with serum and washed before being placed in contact with pneumococci showed no increase in the uptake of bacteria, whereas pneumococci treated in similar fashion and then placed in contact with white cells were readily phagocytized.

Absorption of antiserum with leukocytes failed to alter its properties, whereas absorption with bacteria removed its ability to promote phagocytosis.

Neufeld was to make many important contributions to the bacteriology of the pneumococcus. It was he who discovered the lytic action of bile salts.[29] Prompted by the observations of Koch on the attenuation of the agent of rinderpest by ox bile, Neufeld sought similar effects on a variety of bacterial species, including the pneumococcus. His observation in 1900 of its solubility in bile was a fortuitous find. Two years later he described the quellung reaction.[30] Despite the fact that the quellung reaction was to become ultimately the accepted technique for the capsular typing of pneumococci, Neufeld did not employ it for this purpose for more than a quarter of a century; its first use in the identification of pneumococcal types in humans was not made until 1931.[31] Interestingly, the original work of Neufeld and Händel in identifying pneumococcal types 1 and 2 and the subsequent work of Dochez and Gillespie[32] at the Rockefeller Institute, of Lister[33] in South Africa, and of Cooper and her associates[34] in the New York City Health Department in delineating the additional pneumococcal types recognized during the first three decades of the 20th century were all carried out with other immunologic techniques.

Study of the pneumococcal capsule was to have profound impact on immunology. In 1917 Dochez and Avery published two papers of signal importance, one entitled, "Soluble Substance of Pneumococcus Origin in the Blood and Urine during Lobar Pneumonia,"[35] the other, "The Elaboration of Specific Soluble Substance by Pneumococcus during Growth."[36] So firm at the time was the notion of the association of immunologic activity with protein that the authors wrote the following in the first of these two reports: "The determination of total nitrogen and nitrogen partition on the active substance, obtained by repeated precipitation with acetone and alcohol, shows this substance to be of protein nature or to be associated with protein," even though the material was not destroyed by boiling or by treatment with trypsin. Eight years later, Avery and Morgan[37] were to conclude, "The results of chemical studies previously reported and of those now in progress leave little doubt that the so-called specific soluble substance of Pneumococcus of the three fixed types is in each instance a polysaccharide." Much of the work leading to this conclusion had resulted from the studies of Heidelberger in Avery's laboratory, and, in the same volume of *Journal of Experimental Medicine*, a paper by Avery and Heidelberger[38] described a number of the physiochemical attributes of the capsular polysaccharides of pneumococcal types 1, 2, and 3. Heidelberger[39] was to continue these studies, extending them also to the capsule of Friedländer's bacillus. They were to culminate in a seminal report by Heidelberger and Kendall[40] in 1929 that marked the founding of modern quantitative immunology. Dr. Heidelberger has continued to this very day to use the techniques he developed throughout a long and fruitful career.

Most of the immunologic studies of pneumococcal capsular polysaccharides had been carried out at the Rockefeller Institute with rabbit and with equine antisera; in the course of these studies it had been found that the rabbit, although it produced antibodies to capsular polysaccharide after immunization with whole pneumococci, was refractory to immunization with specific soluble substance. In 1927, Schiemann and Casper[41] reported the immunogenicity of pneumococcal capsular polysaccharide in the mouse; three years later comparable observations with humans were made by Francis and Tillett.[42] These latter studies, extended by Finland and Ruegsegger,[43] opened the way for the development of vaccines of pneumococcal capsular polysaccharides and of comparable antigens from *Neisseria meningitidis* and *Hemophilus influenzae*. Attempts to prevent pneumococcal pneumonia by vaccination had been undertaken initially by Wright[44] and his associates in South Africa in 1911 before the diversity of capsular types was appreciated; the trials of Wright et al., however, failed to establish the efficacy of vaccination. His protégé, Lister, who made many fundamental observations on human immunity to pneumococcal infection, might have demonstrated conclusively the protective value of whole-bacterial pneumococcal vaccines in 1916 had his trials to test their efficacy been structured according to modern epidemiologic requirements.[45] It remained for MacLeod and Heidelberger and their associates, Hodges and Bernhard,[46] to demonstrate unequivocally in 1945 that type-specific pneumococcal infection in man could be prevented by a tetravalent vaccine of capsular polysaccharides and to lay the groundwork for the contemporary vaccine that contains 14 of these capsular antigens.[47]

Although the development of antimicrobial drugs has revolutionized the treatment of bacterial infections, the availability and use of these therapeutic agents have disclosed in an unforeseen way the adaptability of living organisms. The pneumococcus was among the first bacterial species recognized as being capable of developing resistance to an antimicrobial agent. In 1912 Morgenroth and Kaufmann[48] reported what were probably the first observations on the development of resistance in vivo to an antibacterial drug, i.e., Optochin (ethylhydrocuprein), in mice infected with pneumococci and treated with this derivative of quinine. Similar observations on the development of resistance of pneumococci to Optochin in man were described by Moore and Chesney[49] five years later. These findings, however, were made too long a time before the introduction of antibacterial drugs safe and effective for the treatment of humans to be remembered, and their fundamental importance had to be rediscovered at a later date. Only in the past three years have pneumococci

resistant to multiple antimicrobial drugs been recognized.[50] These recent observations have borne out the significance of earlier work and given added
importance to the potential value of the prevention of pneumococcal disease.

Of all the contributions to biology and medicine arising from the study of
the pneumococcus, none has outweighed in importance the elucidation of the
capsular transformation reaction, a discovery that has revolutionized man's
perceptions of the cell and its functions. This discovery had its inception in
the studies of the British bacteriologist Fred Griffith in the third decade of this
century.[51] In studies designed to determine the requirements for the reversion
of noncapsulated avirulent variants of pneumococci to the virulent capsulated
form, Griffith injected living noncapsulated variants derived from one capsular type into mice together with suspensions of heat-killed capsulated variants of the homologous or of a heterologous capsular type. Mice succumbing
to pneumococcal infection yielded capsulated pneumococci of the capsular
type of the heat-killed suspension, whether it was of the parental type from
which the living nonencapsulated variants were derived or of a heterologous
one. These observations, published in 1928, aroused the interest of Avery,
who began a systematic study of the phenomenon in vitro in collaboration
with Dawson, Sia, and Alloway.[52-54] Over the ensuing years, capsular-type
transformation was carried out in the test tube, and a search for the active
principal promoting the reaction culminated in the publication in 1944 by
Avery, MacLeod, and McCarty[55] of the landmark report entitled, "Studies on
the Chemical Nature of the Substance Inducing Transformation of Pneumococcal Types. Induction of Transformation by a Desoxyribonucleic Acid
Fraction Isolated from Pneumococcus Type III." It was the first report of a
biologic activity of a nucleic acid and was to be the cornerstone of the discipline of molecular genetics. Although the significance of these studies was not
fully appreciated at the time of their publication, they are a monument to
Avery, who, with his many talented associates, contributed so much to the
understanding of nature by the persistent and painstaking study of the pneumococcal cell. Through use of DNA-mediated transformation, much additional information concerning the genetics of drug resistance, adaptive en-
zyme formation, capsular synthesis, and cellular separation has been gleaned
by investigators using this fundamental technique.

It is not possible within the time allotted to review all that is known of the
biology of the pneumococcus and of the diseases it causes in humans. Citation
of many contributions of importance has been omitted with regret because of
that limitation, and the lack of reference to them should in no way be considered a denigration of them. Rather, it has been the purpose of this brief historical review to highlight how much of importance can be learned from the
study of a single bacterium and to express the hope that this enormous store of

knowledge will not cease to be a base on which to build for the future as a result of our improved, though still incomplete, ability to deal with pneumococcal infection. Much remains to be learned about the immunology of pneumococcal disease, and we still lack any firm understanding of how the pneumococcus injures the host it invades. There is no problem of greater importance than that relating to our knowledge of pneumococcal infection. From this brief and incomplete summary, it is evident that White's statement of 1938 [1] is still relevant: "The peculiarities of Pneumococcus are yielding a generous return to the investors and speculators who have cast in their resources with its lot, resulting in the accumulation of a store of solid bullion for the scientist and for mankind." The papers that follow will doubtless add to that store.

References

1. White, B. The biology of pneumococcus. Commonwealth Fund, New York, 1938, p. vii–viii.

2. Klebs, E. Beiträge zur Kenntnis der pathogenen Schistomyceten. VII. Die Monadinen. Archiv für experimentelle Pathologie und Pharmakologie (Leipzig) 4: 409–488, 1875.

3. Koch, R. Zur Untersuchung von pathogenen Organismen. Mittheilungen aus dem kaiserlichen Gesundheitsamte (Berlin) 1: 1–48, 1881.

4. Eberth, C. J. Zur Kenntnis der mykotischen Processe. Deutsches Archiv für klinische Medizin (Leipzig) 28: 1–42, 1880.

5. Sternberg, G. M. A fatal form of septicaemia in the rabbit, produced by subcutaneous injection of human saliva. An experimental research. National Board of Health Bulletin 2: 781–783, 1881.

6. Pasteur. Note sur la maladie nouvelle provoquée par la salive d'un enfant mort de la rage. Bulletin de l'Académie de Médicine (Paris) [series 2] 10: 94–103, 1881.

7. Friedländer, C. Ueber die Schizomyceten bei der acuten fibrösen Pneumonie. Virchows Archiv für pathologische Anatomie und Physiologie und für klinische Medizin (Berlin) 87: 319–324, 1882.

8. Friedländer, C. Die Mikrokokken der Pneumonie. Fortschr. Med. 1: 715–733, 1883.

9. Fraenkel, A. Ueber die genuine Pneumonie. Verhandlungen des Congresses für innere Medicin, Dritter Congress 3: 17–31, 1884.

10. Weichselbaum, A. Ueber die Aetiologie der acuten Lungen- und Rippenfellentzündungen. Medizinische Jahrbücher [series 3] 1: 483–554, 1886.

11. Gram, C. Ueber die isolierte Färbung der Schizomyceten in Schnitt- und Trockenpräparaten. Fortschr. Med. 2: 185–189, 1884.

12. Austrian, R. The gram stain and the etiology of lobar pneumonia, an historical note. Bacteriol. Rev. 24: 261–265, 1960.

13. Günther, C. Discussion of Leyden's report. Verhandlungen des Vereins für innere Medicin zu Berlin 2: 123–125, 1882.

14. Leyden, E. Ueber infectiöse Pneumonie. Verhandlungen des Vereins für innere Medicin zu Berlin 2: 121–123, 1882.

15. Talamon. Coccus de la pneumonie. Bulletins de la Société Anatomique de Paris 58: 475–481, 1883.

16. Friedländer, C. Weitere Bemerkungen über Pneumonie-Micrococcen. Fortschr. Med. 2: 333–336, 1884.

17. Osler, W. Infectious (so-called ulcerative) endocarditis. Archives of Medicine 5: 44–68, 1881.

18. Netter. De l'endocardite végétante-ulcéreuse d'origine pneumonique. Archives de Physiologie Normale et Pathologique [series 3] 8: 106–161, 1886.

19. Netter. De la méningite due au pneumocoque (avec ou sans pneumonie). Archives Générales de Médecine [series 7] 19: 257–277, 434–455, 1887.

20. Zaufel, E. Mikroorganismen im Secrete der Otitis media acuta. Prager Medicinische Wochenschrift 12: 225–227, 1887.

21. Weichselbaum, A. Ueber seltenere Localisationen des pneumonischen Virus (*Diplococcus pneumoniae*). Wiener klinische Wochenschrift 1: 659–661, 1888.

22. Sternberg, G. M. The etiology of croupous pneumonia. National Medical Review 7: 175–177, 1897.

23. Fraenkel, A. Bakteriologische Mittheilungen. Zeitschrift für klinische Medicin 10: 401–461, 1885.

24. Klemperer, G., Klemperer, F. Versuche über Immunisirung und Heilung bei der Pneumokokkeninfection. Berliner klinische Wochenschrift 28: 833–835, 869–875, 1891.

25. Neufeld, F., Händel. Weitere Untersuchungen über Pneumokokken Heilsera. III. Mitteilung. Über Vorkommen und Bedeutung atypischer Varietäten des Pneumokokkus. Arbeiten aus dem kaiserlichen Gesundheitsamte 34: 293–304, 1910.

26. Gamaléia, N. Sur l'étiologie de la pneumonie fibrineuse chez l'homme. Annales de l'Institut Pasteur 2: 440–459, 1888.

27. Issaeff, B. Contribution à l'étude de l'immunité acquise contre le pneumocoque. Annales de l'Institut Pasteur 7: 260–279, 1893.

28. Neufeld, F., Rimpau, W. Ueber die Antikörper des Streptokokken- und Pneumokokken-Immunserums. Dtsch. med. Wochenschr. 30: 1458–1460, 1904.

29. Neufeld, F. Ueber eine specifische bakterolytische Wirkung der Galle. Zeitschrift für Hygiene und Infektionskrankheiten (Leipzig) 34: 454–464, 1900.

30. Neufeld, F. Ueber die Agglutination der Pneumokokken und über die Theorieen der Agglutination. Zeitschrift für Hygiene und Infektionskrankheiten 40: 54–72, 1902.

31. Armstrong, R. R. A swift and simple method for deciding pneumococcal "type." Br. Med. J. 1: 214–215, 1931.

32. Dochez, A. R., Gillespie, L. J. A biologic classification of pneumococci by means of immunity reactions. J.A.M.A. 61: 727–730, 1913.

33. Lister, F. S. Specific serological reactions with pneumococci from different sources. Publications of the South African Institute for Medical Research 1 (2): 1–14, 1913.

34. Cooper, G., Rosenstein, C., Walter, A., Peizer, L. The further separation of types among the pneumococci hitherto included in group IV and the development of the therapeutic antisera for these types. J. Exp. Med. 55: 531–554, 1932.

35. Dochez, A. R., Avery, O. T. Soluble substance of pneumococcus origin in the blood and urine during lobar pneumonia. Proc. Soc. Exp. Biol. Med. 14: 126–127, 1917.

36. Dochez, A. R., Avery, O. T. The elaboration of specific soluble substance by pneumococcus during growth. J. Exp. Med. 26: 477–493, 1917.

37. Avery, O. T., Morgan, H. J. Immunological reactions of the isolated carbohydrate and protein of pneumococcus. J. Exp. Med. 42: 347–353, 1925.

38. Avery, O. T., Heidelberger, M. Immunological relationships of cell constituents of pneumococcus. Paper II. J. Exp. Med. 42: 367–376, 1925.

39. Heidelberger, M., Goebel, W. F., Avery, O. T. The soluble specific substance of a strain of Friedländer's bacillus. Paper I. J. Exp. Med. 42: 701–707, 1925.

40. Heidelberger, M., Kendall, F. E. A quantitative study of the precipitin reaction between type III pneumococcus polysaccharide and purified homologous antibody. J. Exp. Med. 50: 809–823, 1929.

41. Schiemann, O., Casper, W. Sind die spezifisch präcipitablen Substanzen der 3 Pneumokokkentypen Haptene? Zeitschrift für Hygiene und Infektionskrankheiten 108: 220–257, 1927.

42. Francis, T., Jr., Tillett, W. S. Cutaneous reactions in pneumonia. The development of antibodies following the intradermal injection of type-specific polysaccharide. J. Exp. Med. 52: 573–585, 1930.

43. Finland, M., Ruegsegger, J. M. Immunization of human subjects with the specific carbohydrates of type III and the related type VIII pneumococcus. J. Clin. Invest. 14: 829–832, 1935.

44. Wright, A. E., Parry Morgan, W., Colebrook, L., Dodgson, R. W. Observations on prophylactic inoculation against pneumococcus infections, and on the results which have been achieved by it. Lancet 1: 1–10, 87-95, 1914.

45. Lister, F. S. An experimental study of prophylactic inoculation against pneumococcal infection in the rabbit and in man. Publications of the South African Institute for Medical Research 1(8): 231–287, 1916.

46. MacLeod, C. M., Hodges, R. G., Heidelberger, M., Bernhard, W. G. Prevention of pneumococcal pneumonia by immunization with specific capsular polysaccharides. J. Exp. Med. 82: 445–465, 1945.

47. Austrian, R., Douglas, R. M., Schiffman, G., Coetzee, A. M., Koornhof, H. J., Hayden-Smith, S., Reid, R. D. W. Prevention of pneumococcal pneumonia by vaccination. Trans. Assoc. Am. Physicians 89: 184–192, 1976.

48. Morgenroth, J., Kaufmann, M. Arzneifestigkeit bei Bakterien (Pneumokokken). Zeitschrift für Immunitätsforschung und experimentelle Therapie 15: 610–624, 1912.

49. Moore, H. F., Chesney, A. M. A study of ethylhydrocuprein (optochin) in the treatment of acute lobar pneumonia. Arch. Intern. Med. 19: 611–682, 1917.

50. Jacobs, M. R., Koornhof, H. J., Robins-Browne, R. M., Stevenson, C. M., Vermaak, Z. A., Freiman, I., Miller, G. B., Whitcomb, M. A., Isaäcson, M., Ward, J. I., Austrian, R. Emergence of multiply resistant pneumococci. N. Engl. J. Med. 299: 735–740, 1978.

51. Griffith, F. The significance of pneumococcal types. J. Hyg. 27: 113–159, 1928.

52. Dawson, M. H. The transformation of pneumococcal types. J. Exp. Med. 51: 99–122, 123–147, 1930.

53. Sia, R. H. P., Dawson, M. H. In vitro transformation of pneumococcal types. II.

The nature of the factor responsible for the transformation of pneumococcal types. J. Exp. Med. 54: 701–710, 1931.

54. Alloway, J. L. Further observations on the use of pneumococcus extracts in effecting transformation of type in vitro. J. Exp. Med. 57: 265–278, 1933.

55. Avery, O. T., MacLeod, C. M., McCarty, M. Studies on the chemical nature of the substance inducing transformation of pneumococcal types. Induction of transformation by a desoxyribonucleic acid fraction isolated from pneumococcus type III. J. Exp. Med. 79: 137–158, 1944.

6

The Current Status of Bacteremic Pneumococcal Pneumonia: Re-evaluation of an Underemphasized Clinical Problem

Although the last quarter century has seen remarkable advances in the prophylaxis and treatment of respiratory infection, pneumonia remains among the leading causes of death in this country. Since the introduction of penicillin, reports of the mortality from pneumococcal bacteremia have varied[1,2] but have placed it as high as 25 per cent. Because of these observations and because there has been no analysis of pneumococcal bacteremia caused by different capsular types since the advent of antibiotics, a study of such infections was undertaken.

The 529 patients included in the investigation were admitted to a 225-bed medical service in the Kings County Hospital, Brooklyn, New York, between 1952 and 1962. Incontravertible evidence of pneumococcal infection was provided in each instance by isolation of pneumococci from the patient's blood, and 99 per cent of the strains recovered were identified by the capsular swelling or "quellung" reaction.

The bacteremic patients can be classified into three groups. There were 455 patients with pneumonia, 47 with pneumonia and an extrapulmonary focus of pneumococcal infection and 27 with meningitis secondary to sinusitis or otitis. The overall mortality for the three groups was 25 per cent. Because of the small size of the two latter groups, however, only the first will be considered in the discussion that follows.

Bacteremic pneumococcal pneumonia resulted in the death of one of every five persons afflicted. The results of treatment are shown in Table 1. In the 438 patients who received antimicrobial therapy, the mortality was 17 per cent. The majority received penicillin, a smaller number tetracycline and the remainder a variety of drugs.

In the subsequent analysis of the results of antimicrobial therapy, the data

Table 1. *Treatment of Pneumococcal Bacteremia*

Treatment	Number	Fatal	% Fatal
Penicillin	338	57	17
Tetracycline	55	10	18
Other	45	8	18
None	17	14	82
Total	455	89	20

will be contrasted with those of Tilghman and Finland,[3] who described a similar group of 480 patients with bacteremic pneumococcal pneumonia treated symptomatically at the Boston City Hospital between 1929 and 1935. The latter group cannot be considered a control in the strict sense of the term. Its use for comparative purposes, however, is dictated by the inadmissibility of withholding antipneumococcal therapy during the course of the present study.

Because of the persisting high death rate associated with pneumococcal bacteremia, answers to the following questions were sought:

(1) Has the death rate from infection caused by different pneumococcal types been affected equally by treatment with antibiotics?

(2) Are certain patients more likely to succumb to pneumococcal infection than others; and, if so, can they be identified?

(3) Are practical measures available that might lead to a lower mortality from pneumococcal disease?

The type of pneumococcus causing infection may play a significant role in prognosis. The six capsular Types I, III, IV, VII, VIII, and XII were responsible for 66 per cent of the pneumococcal pneumonia with bacteremia and for 60 per cent of all deaths from such infection. Figure 1 contrasts the fatality following symptomatic treatment with that after penicillin therapy for each of the six types mentioned and for all capsular types as a group. Although the mortality from Type I pneumococcal infection has declined from 86 per cent to 7 per cent, that following infection with pneumococcus Type III has fallen from 98 per cent only to 48 per cent. Whether the pronounced decline in the death rate from Type I pneumococcal pneumonia with bacteremia is attributable solely to the effect of antimicrobial therapy or, in part, to a reduction in the virulence of the organism cannot be stated with certainty. It is noteworthy, however, that Type I remains the most frequent cause of pneumococcal bacteremia despite the improved prognosis of those infected with it. The persistently high mortality from Type III pneumococcal infection, on the other hand, is consistent with the peculiar biological properties of this capsular

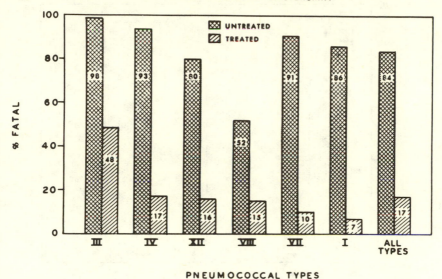

FATALITY IN UNTREATED AND PENICILLIN TREATED
PNEUMOCOCCAL BACTEREMIA

Fig. 1.—Numbers within bars in this and in subsequent figures indicate per cent of fatal cases. Untreated and serum treated cases from Tilghman and Finland[3] unless otherwise indicated.

type. Its resistance to surface phagocytosis and the consequences thereof in the evolution of pulmonary infection, demonstrated so elegantly by Wood and Smith,[4,5] explain, in part at least, the less beneficial effect of antimicrobial treatment in Type III pneumococcal disease. Smaller differences exist in the mortality of infections caused by other capsular types, but it is clear that infections with different types of pneumococci have not been affected to the same degree by antibiotic therapy.

The impact of antibiotics on the outcome of infection in different age groups is shown in Figure 2. Though lowering of mortality is evident in each of the age groups depicted, it is significantly less among those 50 years of age or older. In the two groups of persons under the age of 50, the fatality has been reduced approximately 90 per cent; but, in that comprised of older persons, the reduction has been about 65 per cent.

The presence or absence of pre-existing complicating illness also plays an important role in prognosis in bacteremic pneumococcal pneumonia. Figure 3

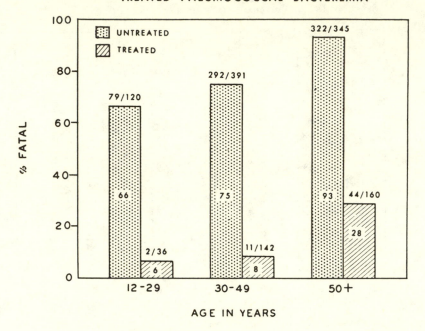

Fig. 2.—Denominator of fraction above bar indicates total number of cases, numerator number of fatal cases. Data for untreated cases include those of Bullowa.[12]

shows that antibiotic therapy has brought about a lesser improvement in the recovery rate of those with complicating illness than in that of those who lack it. The difference in mortality between the two groups is comparable to that observed in the recovery rates of persons under 50 and of those 50 years of age or older.

If the three factors of infecting pneumococcal type, age of the patient and the presence or absence of complicating illness are considered together, it is possible to delineate an element of the population at high risk of death from pneumococcal bacteremia. Figure 4 relates these three factors and indicates that more than half of all deaths from pneumococcal bacteremia are caused by pneumococcus Types I, III, IV, VII, VIII, and XII. Two-thirds of these deaths occur in persons 50 years of age or older with complicating illness. If bacteremic infections with any of the same six types in persons under 50 with complicating illness and in those 50 or older with or without complicating disease are combined, these categories account for nearly three-fifths of all deaths from pneumococcal bacteremia.

It is pertinent now to ask whether or not all bacteremic patients treated with antibiotics are benefited significantly by such therapy. To answer this question, three groups of patients will be considered: those treated symptomatically, those treated with serum and those treated with penicillin. If the per cent of survivors in each group is plotted against the duration of illness in days, a curve is obtained for each group which is shown in Figure 5. Although the three curves diverge widely after the fifth day of illness, there is striking similarity among them prior to this time. Stated differently, antipneumococcal therapy has little or no effect on the outcome of infection among those destined, at the onset of illness, to die within 5 days. Although the scale of the curves may make the number of deaths in this period seem insignificant, 60 per cent of all deaths among all patients treated with penicillin occurred in the 5 days following the onset of illness. In other words, by the time antimicrobial

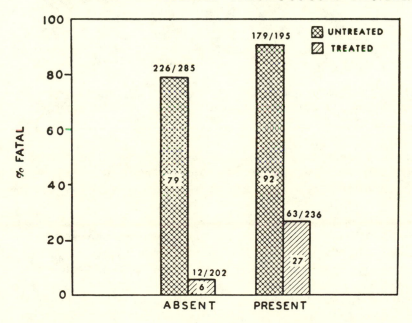

Fig. 3.—The data include all patients treated with antibiotics.

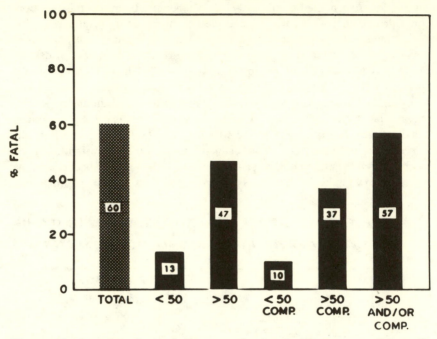

Fig. 4.—Numbers along abscissa indicate ages of patients in different groups. "Comp." designates pneumococcal infection complicated by pre-existing illness such as heart, liver, endocrine disease, *etc.*

therapy was instituted, and even when it was begun on occasion on the first day of illness, the patient had passed "the physiologic point of no return," and no treatment directed solely against the infecting organism could preserve his life.

In the light of the foregoing data, it appears unlikely that the prognosis in pneumococcal infection can be improved further by antimicrobial therapy. Penicillin is rapidly bactericidal, non-toxic, and pneumococcal mutants resistant to it do not arise during therapy. A more favorable outlook following treatment can be anticipated only when the physiologic derangements brought about by infection are better understood and specific measures are devised to correct them. Until then, prophylactic measures would appear to offer the most likely means of reducing further the mortality from pneumococcal bacteremia and from pneumococcal infection.

Purified pneumococcal capsular polysaccharides are excellent antigens in man. Convincing evidence of their efficacy in reducing the incidence of pneumococcal infection caused by several capsular types has been provided by the well controlled studies of MacLeod and his co-workers.[6] Other studies have shown that a satisfactory response to each of six different capsular polysaccharides injected simultaneously may be expected;[7] and the observations of Heidelberger[8] have demonstrated that half maximal levels of antibody evoked by a single immunizing injection may be present 5 years later. That older persons respond satisfactorily to pneumococcal vaccines has been demonstrated by Kaufman,[9] whose results in a controlled study involving 10,000 persons over 50 years of age showed a 90 per cent reduction in the immunized group in the rate of infection and of bacteremia caused by pneumococcal types included in the vaccine.

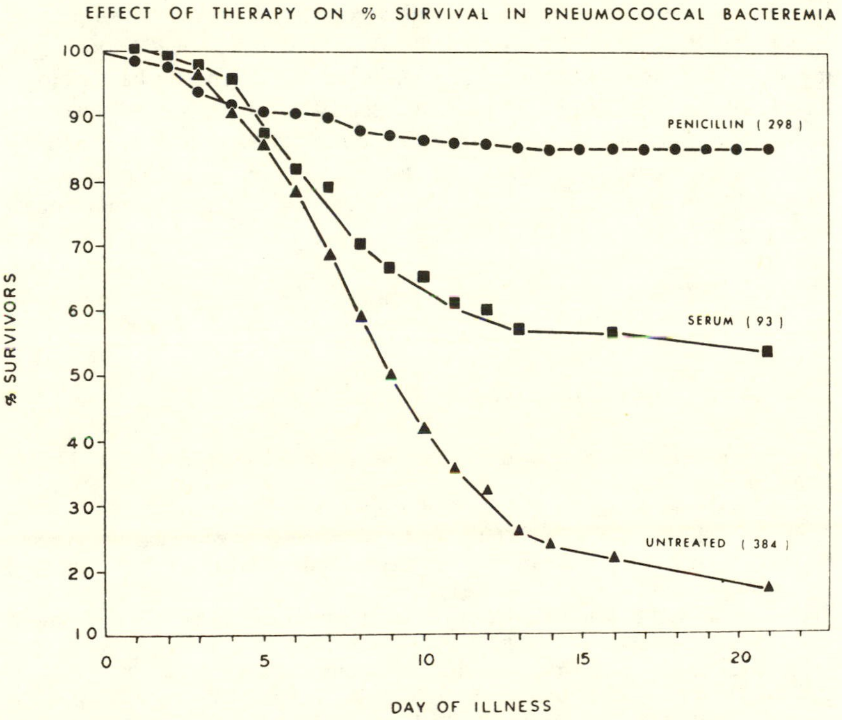

EFFECT OF THERAPY ON % SURVIVAL IN PNEUMOCOCCAL BACTEREMIA

Fig. 5.—Numbers in parentheses indicate size of each group of patients. Serum treated patients include only pneumococcal Types I and II.[3]

On the basis of the available evidence, it is concluded that it is entirely feasible to immunize a definable group of the population known to be at high risk of death following infection with identifiable pneumococcal types. This group resembles closely that at high risk of death from influenza viral infection.

Finally, it may be asked whether or not a program of immunization of the type described is worthwhile. "Pneumonia and influenza" constitutes today the only category of infectious disease among the ten leading causes of death in the United States. In 1961, a year in which influenza was not epidemic, there were 55,175 deaths classified in this category,[10] and the death rate from these causes for the population as a whole was more than 100 times that from poliomyelitis. The Bureau of Vital Statistics of the United States[11] projects an increase in the number of persons over 55 years of age from 28,500,000 in 1955 to 46,000,000 in 1980. If it is worthwhile to invest large sums in the palliation and cure of neoplastic and of cardiovascular diseases, which affect most heavily this segment of the population, it seems reasonable to utilize available knowledge to reduce the morbidity and mortality resulting from one of the most common bacterial infections in our society. To provide essential epidemiologic data, it will be necessary to make pneumococcal typing sera available once again and to reinstitute the diagnostic bacteriologic techniques for identification of pneumococcus which have been all but completely abandoned by the medical profession. With these measures and the utilization of knowledge already extant concerning immunization, it should be possible to prevent 10,000 to 15,000 deaths a year from pneumococcal infection.

References

1. Finland, M.: Treatment of pneumonia and other serious infections. N. Eng. J. Med., 263: 207–221, 1960.

2. Dowling, H. F. and Lepper, M. H.: The effect of antibiotics (Penicillin, Aureomycin, and Terramycin) on the fatality rate and incidence of complications in pneumococcic pneumonia. A comparison with other methods of therapy. Am. J. Med. Sc., 222: 396–403, 1951.

3. Tilghman, R. C. and Finland, M.: Clinical significance of bacteremia in pneumococcic pneumonia. Arch. Int. Med., 59: 602–619, 1937.

4. Wood, W. B., Jr. and Smith, M. R.: The inhibition of surface phagocytosis by the capsular "Slime Layer" of pneumococcus Type III. J. Exp. Med., 90: 85–96, 1949.

5. Wood, W. B., Jr. and Smith, M. R.: Host-parasite relationships in experimental pneumonia due to pneumococcus Type III. J. Exp. Med., 92: 85–100, 1950.

6. MacLeod, C. M., Hodges, R. G., Heidelberger, M., and Bernhard, W. G.: Pre-

vention of pneumococcal pneumonia by immunization with specific capsular polysaccharides. J. Exp. Med., 82: 445–465, 1945.

7. Heidelberger, M., MacLeod, C. M. and Di Lapi, M.: The human antibody response to simultaneous injection of six specific polysaccharides of pneumococcus. J. Exp. Med., 88: 369–372, 1948.

8. Heidelberger, M.: Persistence of antibodies in man after immunization, in The Nature and Significance of the Antibody Response. A. M. Pappenheimer, Jr., Editor. Columbia University Press, New York, 1953, pp. 90–101.

9. Kaufman, P.: Pneumonia in old age. Arch. Int. Med., 79: 518–531, 1947.

10. Advance Report, Vital Statistics of the United States, 1961. Final natality and mortality statistics. National Vital Statistics Division, U.S. Dept. of Health, Education and Welfare, Public Health Service, November, 1962.

11. Statistical Abstract of the United States, 1958. U.S. Dept. of Commerce, Bureau of the Census, 79th Annual Edition, U.S. Government Printing Office, Washington, D.C., 1958, p. 6.

12. Bullowa, J. G. M.: The Management of the Pneumonias. Oxford University Press, New York, 1937, p. 71.

7

Prevention of Pneumococcal Pneumonia by Vaccination

ROBERT AUSTRIAN, ROBERT M. DOUGLAS,
GERALD SCHIFFMAN, ALBERT M. COETZEE,
HENDRIK J. KOORNHOF, STANLEY HAYDEN-
SMITH AND ROBERT D. W. REID

In a study reported thirteen years ago to this Association,[1] it was found that the overall mortality of bacteremic pneumococcal pneumonia treated with penicillin was 17 per cent. In that same study, it was observed also that the fatality rate in persons 50 years of age and older and in individuals with a variety of chronic systemic illnesses exceeded 25 per cent. Examination of survival curves revealed that 60 per cent of all deaths occurring in individuals with bacteremic pneumococcal pneumonia treated with penicillin occurred in the first five days following the onset of illness and resulted apparently from early irreversible physiologic injury which was unaffected by specific antimicrobial therapy. Because the precise nature of the physiologic derangements resulting from pneumococcal infection were unknown at that time and are still unknown, prophylaxis appeared to offer the sole means available to reduce the significant number of illnesses and deaths in those at high risk of a fatal outcome. For these reasons, steps were undertaken to redevelop polyvalent vaccines of pneumococcal capsular polysaccharides, which had been shown previously to be effective by MacLeod et al.[2] in an epidemic of pneumonia in a military population during World War II.

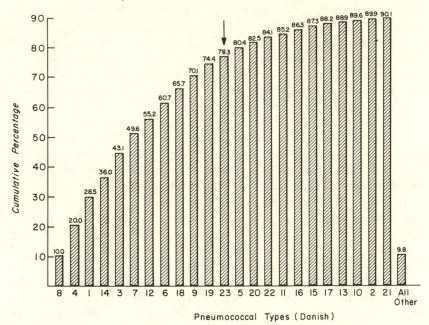

Fig. 1.—Cumulative incidence of pneumococcal types isolated from blood cultures of patients with bacteremic infection in ten American cities, 1967–1975.

To achieve the desired goal, it was necessary to obtain a variety of data. These included:

(1) identification of the pneumococcal types most often responsible for bacteremic infection in man,

(2) demonstration of the safety and antigenicity of the vaccines to be employed,

(3) determination of the efficacy of the components of polyvalent vaccines in preventing type-specific pneumococcal infection, and

(4) assessment of the impact of the vaccines on the total burden of pneumonia in populations under scrutiny with the passage of time.

Eighty-six pneumococcal capsular types* are now known, but they exhibit

---

*The nomenclature of pneumococcal types is that employed in the labeling of typing sera from the Statens Seruminstitut, Copenhagen, Denmark (Bull. Wld. Hlth. Org. 23: 5, 1960). In 1985, the number of types recognized is eighty-four.

marked differences in their invasiveness in man. To determine which types should be included in contemporary vaccines, monitoring of strains isolated from blood cultures in hospitals in ten American communities widely distributed throughout the country was initiated in 1967. Since that time, 3644 isolates from such cultures have been typed. The distribution of their types is plotted cumulatively in Figure 1. From the figure, it may be seen that the cumulative incidence of bacteremic pneumococcal infections observed in this sample yields a semilogarithmic curve when successive types are ranked in order of decreasing frequency. Six types account for approximately half, twelve types for three-quarters and eighteen types for seven-eighths of these infections. Although vaccines of six capsular polysaccharides have been given previously to man, this number of antigens appeared too small to be suitable in the light of more recent findings; and vaccines containing twelve to fourteen capsular polysaccharides were ultimately developed.

To determine the safety and antigenicity of pneumococcal vaccines, the capsular polysaccharides of 15 individual types, types 1, 2, 3, 4, 5, 6, 7, 8, 9, 12, 14, 18, 19, 23 and 25, were prepared commercially; and all were tested for antigenicity in volunteers, the majority in doses ranging from 5 μg to 1000 μg. The safety of monovalent vaccines was readily demonstrable; and a dose of 50 μg, that used earlier by MacLeod and his associates,[2] was found to be a suitable one of each capsular antigen. The individual polysaccharides were then combined into polyvalent formulations. Figure 2 shows the fold increases in the geometric mean levels of antibodies to each of the thirteen antigens in a tridecavalent pneumococcal vaccine six weeks after its administration to eleven volunteers. They range between 6.3 and 25.8 fold. With time, the levels decline somewhat; but, as found by Heidelberger and his associates,[3] they persist at a third to a half their peak values two to three years after a single injection. The safety of a dodecavalent vaccine administered to more than 6000 individuals under the supervision of Dr. Marvin Freid at the Kaiser Permanente Medical Center in San Francisco is attested by the data in Figure 3. Although reactions to polyvalent formulations of pneumococcal capsular polysaccharides are somewhat more frequent than are those to monovalent ones, their frequency and severity are far less than those to typhoid vaccine. Approximately 40 per cent of individuals receiving simultaneously twelve capsular polysaccharides had some discomfort or pain at the site of injection, 35 per cent developed local erythema lasting for a day, and 3.4 per cent experienced slight elevation of temperature of similar duration. Sixty per cent of the recipients of the vaccine experienced no untoward reaction whatever.

The safety and antigenicity of several polyvalent pneumococcal vaccines having been demonstrated, it remained to assess their efficacy in preventing pneumococcal illness. To this end, several field trials of such vaccines were

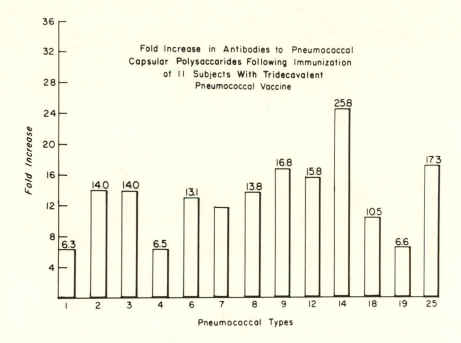

Fig. 2.—Fold increases in levels of antibodies to type-specific pneumococcal capsular polysaccharides six weeks following injection of tridecavalent pneumococcal vaccine in a dose of 50 μg of each antigen.

designed. When it was learned seven years ago that pneumonia was still epidemic among gold mining novices in South Africa, bacteriologic surveillance to determine its cause was initiated at the East Rand Proprietary Mine near Johannesburg in 1970. It was soon found that pneumococcus was the prevalent cause of pneumonia as it had been ever since the discovery of gold and the opening of the mines on the reef. The attack rate of putative pneumococcal pneumonia among men coming to work for the first time in the mine was found to be 90 per 1000 man-years exposure. Such a population provided an ideal one for the testing of pneumococcal vaccines, and the participation of its members was enlisted after seeking and obtaining their consent.

Three trials were conducted, involving 12,000 young adult males, mostly from Malawi and Mozambique. The trials were structured so that men were assigned from a table of random numbers to receive either a polyvalent pneumococcal vaccine, Group A meningococcal vaccine or a saline placebo. In the

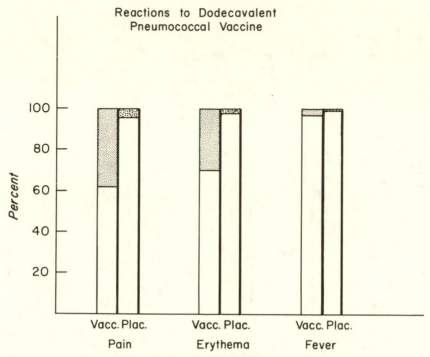

Fig. 3.—Incidence of local and systemic reactions in 6172 recipients of dodecavalent pneumococcal vaccine containing 50 μg each of the capsular polysaccharides of types 1, 3, 4, 6, 7, 8, 9, 12, 14, 18, 19 and 23 and in 6105 recipients of saline placebo. Clear areas indicate absence of reaction.

first trial, a hexavalent vaccine containing the capsular polysaccharides of pneumococcal types 1, 3, 4, 7, 8 and 12 was employed. In the two subsequent trials, a tridecavalent vaccine containing, in addition, the capsular polysaccharides of types 2, 6, 9, 14, 18, 19 and 25 was used. The dose of each antigen was 50 μg. In the results to be presented, comparable data from the three trials have been combined where relevant.

Figure 4 depicts the incidence of putative pneumococcal pneumonia and/or pneumococcal bacteremia occurring later than two weeks after injection among 1493 recipients of tridecavalent pneumococcal vaccine, 1527 recipients of Group A meningococcal vaccine and 1480 recipients of a saline placebo. The efficacy of the vaccine is 78.5 per cent, and the probability of the result's occurring by chance, determined by the chi square test, is less than one in ten thousand. Protection against putative infection with six individual

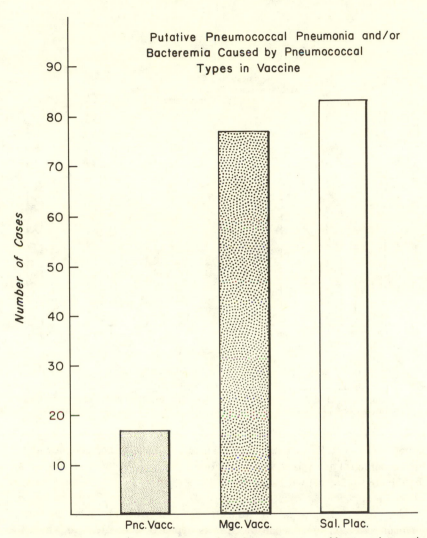

Fig. 4.—Putative pneumococcal pneumonia and/or pneumococcal bacteremia associated with capsular types in tridecavalent vaccine occurring later than two weeks after injection. There were 17 cases in pneumococcal vaccinees, 77 in meningococcal vaccinees and 83 in recipients of placebo. The difference between the pneumococcal vaccinees and the two control cohorts is statistically significant ($X^2 = 46.3$; $p < 0.0001$).

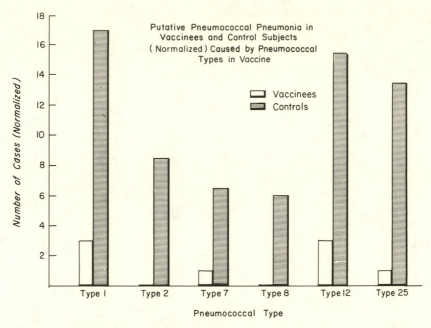

Fig. 5.—Putative pneumococcal pneumonia associated with individual types in tri-decavalent pneumococcal vaccine occurring later than two weeks after injection in 1493 pneumococcal vaccinees and in 3007 control subjects. The numbers of illnesses in controls have been normalized by dividing by two.

types included in the vaccine which occurred with sufficient frequency to permit meaningful analysis is shown in Figure 5. All differences are significant by the chi square test with a p value for type 7 of 0.038 and of less than 0.01 for the remainder.

Unequivocal demonstration of the efficacy of the vaccines in the prevention of bacteremic pneumococcal infection is depicted in Figure 6 in which the data from all three trials are combined. The vaccines were 82.3 per cent effective in preventing pneumococcal bacteremia caused by types included in them. Three pneumococcal types not included in the vaccines accounted for more than half the remaining bacteremic infections, types 5, 45 and 46, the latter two of which are rarely found in the United States. Of the 10 bacteremic infections occurring in pneumococcal vaccinees and caused by types in the vaccine, eight were infections with pneumococcus type 1. Subsequent analysis of the type 1 antigen in the vaccine by radioimmunoassay showed that it

contained 9 μg rather than the purported 50 μg of type I pneumococcal capsular polysaccharide per dose. Although the vaccine provided 72 per cent protection against type I pneumococcal bacteremia at a high level of statistical
significance, it is probable that the dose of type I antigen administered is a
borderline one for the immunization of adults and that better results might
have been achieved had the dose of antigen been higher.

Throughout the course of these investigations, the question has been raised
repeatedly whether or not disease eliminated by prevention of infection with
selected pneumococcal types would lead to its replacement by illness caused
by other pneumococcal types. Figure 7 illustrates the incidence of radiologically confirmed pneumonia occurring later than two weeks following
injection, irrespective of cause, in pneumococcal vaccinees and in the two
control cohorts two years after the start of the trial. The attack rate of radi-

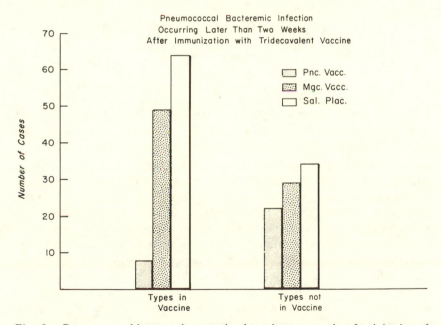

Fig. 6.—Pneumococcal bacteremia occurring later than two weeks after injection of
pneumococcal vaccinees, meningococcal vaccinees and recipients of placebo (combined data from trials of hexavalent and tridecavalent pneumococcal vaccines). There
were 10 bacteremias caused by types in the vaccines in pneumococcal vaccinees, 49 in
meningococcal vaccinees and 64 in recipients of placebo. The difference between
pneumococcal vaccinees and controls is significant ($X^2 = 34.8$; p < 0.0001).

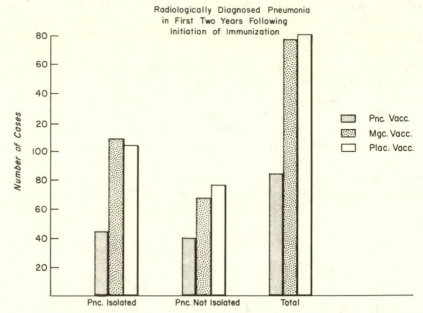

Fig. 7.—Radiologically confirmed pneumonia irrespective of cause, occurring later than two weeks following injection in pneumococcal vaccinees, meningococcal vaccinees and recipients of placebo in first two years following initiation of field trials of tridecavalent pneumococcal vaccine. All differences between pneumococcal vaccinees and control cohorts are statistically significant (p values < 0.0001).

ologically confirmed pneumonia in pneumococcal vaccinees has been reduced by slightly more than half, and it has been shown that this reduction has been maintained over a period of a year in a closed population into which new potentially susceptible subjects were being introduced. Whether or not the reduction would be maintained indefinitely cannot be ascertained at this time. It is not unlikely, however, that the introduction of a virulent strain of influenza virus might alter the picture, temporarily at least, as was suggested during earlier trials of whole bacterial pneumococcal vaccines in South Africa. Over the period of observation, however, even the two most prevalent pneumococcal types not included in the vaccine showed no increasing tendency to attack those protected against infection with other types included in the vaccine.

In summary, polyvalent vaccines of pneumococcal capsular polysaccharides have been shown to be safe, antigenic and at least 78.5 per cent effective in providing protection against type-specific putative pneumococcal pneumonia. Their efficacy in preventing bacteremic infection with the same organisms was

82.3 per cent. Their licensure is anticipated within the next year and they should provide useful prophylactic agents for administration to adults at higher than average risk of a fatal outcome of pneumococcal infection. These include individuals 50 years of age and older, those with a variety of chronic systemic illness, individuals with anatomic or functional asplenia and those with sicklemia. Were the number of antigens in the vaccine to be increased from 12 to 20, bringing the total dose of polysaccharides to 1 mgm, and were the vaccine to be used widely, the prospect of largely eliminating the half million pneumococcal pneumonias estimated to occur annually in the adult population of this country would appear to be a realizable one.

(From the Department of Research Medicine, the University of Pennsylvania School of Medicine, Philadelphia, Pennsylvania; the Department of Microbiology, SUNY Downstate Medical Center, Brooklyn, New York; the South African Institute for Medical Research, Johannesburg, South Africa; and the Hospital of the East Rand Proprietary Mine, Boksburg, South Africa.)

Acknowledgments: I am indebted to the following investigators for their contributions to several facets of the pneumococcal vaccine program. Surveillance of pneumococcal types responsible for bacteremic infections: Drs. H. W. Beaty, H. P. Bernheimer, T. C. Eickhoff, M. Finland, M. Hamburger, D. Ivler, W. I. Metzger, M. H. D. Smith, B. Tempest and E. Wolinsky. Field trials of pneumococcal vaccines: Drs. J. H. S. Gear, J. G. D. Laing, P. Smit, and C. H. Wyndham of South Africa; Dr. M. Freid, Kaiser Permanente Medical Center, San Francisco. Immunologic studies: Dr. M. J. Bonner.

References

1. Austrian, R.: The current status of bacteremic pneumococcal pneumonia. Reevaluation of an underemphasized clinical problem. Trans. Assoc. Am. Phys. 76: 117, 1963.

2. MacLeod, C. M., Hodges, R. G., Heidelberger, M., and Bernhard, W. G.: Prevention of pneumococcal pneumonia by immunization with specific capsular polysaccharides. J. Exp. Med. 82: 445, 1945.

3. Heidelberger, M., di Lapi, M. M., Siegel, M., and Walter, A. W.: Persistence of antibodies in human subjects injected with pneumococcal polysaccharides. J. Immunol. 65: 535, 1950.

8

Of Gold and Pneumococci: A History of Pneumococcal Vaccines in South Africa

The history of the prevention of pneumococcal pneumonia is inextricably intertwined with that of the South African gold mining industry. I have chosen this topic for the Jeremiah Metzger Lecture for several reasons. They include the long-standing interest of this Association in respiratory disease, the role that several members of this society have played in the evolution of pneumococcal vaccines and the recently recognized emergence of pneumococci resistant to multiple antimicrobial drugs which gives added impetus to the utilization of pneumococcal vaccines as the latter become available once again to physicians.

The pneumococcus was discovered in 1880 almost simultaneously by Sternberg[61] in the United States and by Pasteur[56] in France. Six years later, in 1886, its predominant role as the cause of lobar pneumonia in man was established by Weichselbaum[63] in a classic paper which resolved the bitter polemic between Friedländer and Fraenkel over the etiology of this scourge of mankind.[5] The same year marked the opening of the Witwatersrand gold fields in the Transvaal and the founding of Johannesburg,[29] events which were to have a profound effect on the efforts of the medical profession to control the ravages of pneumococcal infection.

The opening of the world's richest gold field was followed by an explosive development of the mining industry. The profitable mining of gold depended then, as it does now, on an abundant supply of cheap labor; and as the industry expanded, so did its labor force. Between 1893, the earliest year for which statistics are available,[11] and 1899, the year of the outbreak of the Boer War, the number of native Africans employed on the mines rose from 25,049 to 111,697.[29] "The system by which these men were brought to the mines was a somewhat rough-and-ready one," writes Cartwright in his book *Doctors of the Mines*, "and it is perhaps best not to inquire too closely into the methods employed by the recruiters who delivered the first 'kaffirs,' as they were then called, at so much per head."[11] Many suffered from malnutrition, including scurvy, and became ill during the arduous journey from their kraals to the mine compounds on the Reef, where, if they survived, they worked for periods of six to nine months before returning to their homes. The system of employment for limited periods, which has been maintained by the mining industry, resulted in a constant turn-over of the labor force and the continuous introduction of new susceptible individuals into the mine compounds.

Respiratory disease was recognized early among the native miners. In 1894, a paper entitled "Acute Specific Rhinitis" was read before the Transvaal Medical Society describing an epidemic of at least one hundred cases characterized by "purulent discharge from the nostrils and, in a large majority of cases, Pneumonia." Fifteen died, of whom nine were autopsied. Four had pneumonia and three purulent meningitis, whereas one died a toxemic death with no localized findings. In most, there was striking evidence of purulent sinusitis. In 1899, Brodie, Rogers and Hamilton described a similar epidemic among men recruited from Mozambique.[10] The severity of the illness is apparent from the following quotation: "One batch of ninety-three emaciated Kaffirs arrived in the beginning of July, when the temperature, except for a few hours during the day, persisted below freezing point; a fortnight later sixteen were working, and some of these were ailing; altogether of this batch eight died." Among a larger group of eight hundred, twenty-six were autopsied and the tissues of fifteen were cultured. From seven, capsulated diplococci staining by Gram's method and pathogenic for rabbits were isolated. The authors concluded that pneumococcus was responsible for the illnesses observed and that it caused sinusitis, meningitis and pneumonia. Although no work was done on immunity, they expressed the hope that a serum could be prepared which might be efficient in cases of ordinary "pneumonia" occuring in Europeans. "In excuse for these shortcomings of our contribution," they wrote, "we can only say that the present work was carried out in the spare time snatched from our private practices. . . ." As an aside, it may be of interest to those present that the "Transactions of the American Climatological Association for 1898" were reviewed extensively in the succeeding volume of the South African Medical Journal,[28] publication of which was suspended a month later "by reason of the dislocation of affairs in South Africa;" i.e., the Boer War.

Mining of gold came largely to a halt during the war and was gradually resumed after the signing of the Treaty of Vereeniging in 1902. Two years later, Waldon[62] cited again the importance of pneumonia in the native compounds. "Pneumonia in endemic form with epidemic outbreaks is certainly one of the scourges of mining compounds in this country. . . . The mortality of the disease is so high that humanitarian reasons on behalf of the native, and economic reasons on behalf of the employer of labour call for active measures."

"The native while living under conditions found in the average compound undoubtedly seems to be remarkably easy prey to the trouble, and so long as native labour is used in the mines, which I hope will be as long as the mines are working, it is probable that Pneumonia will be commoner among them than in any other community of equal numbers. But if the disease is a necesary evil to some extent it certainly is not to the extent that has prevailed up to the present." Waldron advocated huts admitting sunlight with concrete floors that could be scrubbed and control of expectoration. Three years later a report on pneumonia at the Premier Mine noted the attack rate over a fifteen month period to have been 8/1000/month and the death rate 2/1000/month.[45] The economic aspect of preventable deaths was assessed the following year by George D. Maynard, who recorded the total loss from deaths and sickness resulting from enteric fever, diarrhoea and dysentery, tuberculosis and pneumonia to equal 3,000,000 pounds per year. He observed with some asperity that the government worries about deaths in cattle but not in man.[38]

The continuing concern over both the morbidity and mortality of pneumonia, especially in so-called Tropicals, native Africans from north of latitude 22° South, prompted the heads of several mining companies to seek at least partial solutions to this problem. In February, 1911, Sir Julius Wernher, Chairman of the Central Mining and Investment Corporation in London, consulted with Sir Almroth Wright, who had achieved renown as the developer of typhoid vaccine.[11] I heard first of Sir Almroth from my father in recounting his trip to England in 1912. He was traveling abroad with a male contemporary, as befitted those times; and, having known Sir William Osler as a medical student, he telephoned Osler during a visit to Oxford to pay his respects. He was bidden forthwith to visit 13 Norham Gardens; and, when he demurred on the ground that he was traveling with a companion, Osler's immediate rejoinder was: "That's all right, Austrian, I'll introduce her to Lady Osler as Mrs. Austrian and she'll never know the difference!" So both travelers went to the Osler abode, where, in the course of the conversation, Osler opined that father should meet Sir Almroth Wright. Again father demurred, this time on the ground that Sir Almroth was too busy a man to take time for such a visit. As father left to return to London, Osler came running out of the house with an unsealed letter addressed to Sir Almroth, which father was asked to deliver. As the hack pulled away from the curb, Osler called out "Oh, Austrian, you may read the letter." Ensconced on the train, father took the missive from its envelope and read: "Dear Sir Almroth, This is to introduce Austrian, who does not want to meet you." Unfortunately, I have no recollection of what transpired at the meeting initiated in this typical Oslerian manner.

Wright, who was elected to honorary membership in this Association in 1917, must have been a most extraordinary man. I can find no record that he ever attended one of our meetings. Born of a Swedish mother and Irish father, his biographers attribute his polemical temperament to his sire.[13,15] Described variously by acquaintances as resembling "Tenniel's illustration of the Lion in Alice Through the Looking Glass"[25] and as having "had the narrowest squeak possible from being acromegalic,"[15] he engaged frequently in controversy both in the medical arena and in the larger world as a vocal opponent of women's suffrage. He was a close acquaintance of that active opponent of vaccination, George Bernard Shaw, and was the model for Sir Colenso Ridgeon, the hero of Shaw's play, "The Doctor's Dilemma." Wright is alleged to have walked out of a performance of the play.[13]

Wright's first major controversy was with the British army and with Karl Pearson, the statistician, over the efficacy of typhoid vaccine. Wright seems to have had an antipathy for the mathematical approach to science. In a review of his book, *Principles of Microscopy* published in 1906, the following comment appears: "Sir A. E. Wright labours under heavy self-imposed difficulties. He always seeks to avoid a mathematical sign, the use of which, as a substitute for speech, can be defended, he says, only in the case of the inarticulate classes of the learned. He ignores the fact that speech, whether in sound or black and white, is as much sign as mathematical expression is sign, and nothing like so accurate."[8] It is of interest that the polemic over the use of typhoid vaccine by the British army was resolved largely by Lord Haldane, then Minister of War, who believed in its utility and had succeeded in getting Wright his knighthood, as indicated in the following letter:

"Dear Wright: We must have your Typhoid Prophylactic for the Army but I have failed to convince the head man in the Army Medical Service of this. I have therefore got to build you up as a Public Great Man: the first thing is to make you a knight. You won't like it, but it has to be. Haldane."[15]

In his 1911 meeting with Wernher, Wright indicated he was now working on the problem of pneumonia and suggested that it might be worthwhile to study the utility of vaccines in South Africa. The eventual outcome of the meeting was that Wright agreed to go to South Africa for six months with a stipend of R 2000 a month to be paid by the Witwatersrand Native Labour Association.[11] Wright arrived in South Africa with R. W. Dodgson and W. Parry Morgan in September, 1911; and they were joined shortly thereafter by Leonard Colebrook. They were assisted by several local physicians in Johannesburg, including F. Spencer Lister, of whom more will be said presently.

The work of Wright and his associates in South Africa may be divided into two areas, that dealing with the pharmaco-therapy of pneumonia with Optochin and that relating to the therapeutic and prophylactic use of pneumococcal vaccines.[65,66] Wright had a very clear perception of antimicrobial agents as distinct from antiseptics, which he viewed correctly as protoplasmic poisons. He was familiar with Morgenroth's work in Germany on the experimental use of Optochin in pneumococcal infection,[44] and he studied the pneumococcidal power of the drug in the sera both of healthy Africans and of eight ill with pneumonia. This investigation was abandoned, however, when Morgenroth cabled Wright to advise him of the toxicity of the drug to the optic nerve.

The most noteworthy aspect of Wright's report of his work, however, is his philosophic discourse on the "problem as to what logical methods ought to come into application in enquiries into the efficacy of therapeutic agents" and his "discussion of the question as to whether we ought in this enquiry to bring into application the method of experiential or that of statistical evaluation." [65,66] Time does not permit an analysis of Wright's views; suffice it to say that they provoked the following brisk response from Major Greenwood, then statistician to the Lister Institute of Preventive Medicine:[24]

"Sir Almroth Wright has recently enunciated various methodological conclusions of far-reaching importance, and I propose to attempt an examination of their scope and validity. It will, perhaps, appear an act of presumption on my part to enter the lists with so redoubtable an adversary, but some justification is afforded by the following circumstances. Sir Almroth Wright has satisfied himself that the application of statistical or biometric processes to medical problems cannot yield trustworthy results. . . ."

"The present topic is highly controversial; I have endeavoured to bear in mind the words of Cromwell: 'I beseech you, in the bowels of Christ, think it possible you may be mistaken.' If, however, in the heat of conflict or the vanity of authorship I have used any expression unseemly in one discussing a vast and complex subject with an older and abler man, I beg that the offense may be attributed to carelessness, not to malice." Greenwood proceeded to analyse statistically the reliability of Wright's opsonic index, using for part of the task slides prepared in Wright's laboratory by "Mr. Alexander Fleming." His paper, which attests to the utility of the mathematical approach, ends with the following quotation: ". . . it is pleasing for the advocates of medicostatistical methods to read the tribute of Sir William Osler paid in words which may fitly conclude this paper: 'Karl Pearson's new iatromathematical school of medicine has done good work in making the profession more careful about its facts as well as its figures.'"

As stated earlier, Wright and his coworkers carried out studies to evaluate both the therapeutic and prophylactic effects of pneumococcal vaccines, some of which had been prepared in London and others in Johannesburg. Although two types of pneumococci had been described a year earlier by Neufeld and Händel,[46] the vaccines employed in Johannesburg contained strains of one or more undefined capsular types. Wright attempted to determine by use of the opsonic index the therapeutic dose of pneumococcal vaccine to be employed but was thwarted by the failure of the sera of most patients to react with the strains of pneumococci used in the laboratory, and vaccine therapy proved ineffectual. He turned, therefore, to a study of the prophylactic value of vaccines.

On October 4, 1911, a series of six mass inoculation experiments was begun. To establish that the pneumonia under scrutiny was indeed pneumococcal in origin, blood cultures were obtained from 390 Tropical Natives with pneumonia; and pneumococci were recovered from 99 (25.4%), of whom 56 per cent died. It seems curious that, in subsequent trials of vaccines, the limited bacteriologic data obtained were derived largely from lung punctures or from expectorated sputums; for the efficacy or lack thereof of vaccine could have been established unequivocally from the study of bacteremic infection alone. These initial inoculation experiments differed in a variety of ways including the dosages and numbers of injections administered, the locales of the trials and the proportions of control subjects.[65,66] Wright did not stay for their completion, placing them in the hands of Parry Morgan. He departed from South Africa in the spring of 1912, but not before lecturing in Cape Town. His remarks are recorded in the South African Medical Record of March 19, 1912,[64] and provoked both complimentary and critical editorial comment:[19] "The tone of his discourse is indicated by one of his sentences. 'Indeed one can hardly suggest a disease which is not bacteriological.' Now it is surely outdoing Metschnikoff himself to attribute all atheroma to bacteria, and also all heart disease. Then, again, how can all dyspepsia and all rheumatoid arthritis be due to pyorrhoea alveolaris, when these diseases may frequently occur in patients whose buccal cavities are pictures of pink perfection?"

The trials, which included approximately 50,000 vaccines, were completed in 1912 and the results published in the Lancet in January, 1914.[65] Wright concluded from his analysis of the trials that "the comparative statistics which have been set forth above testify. . . . in every case to a reduction in the incidence-rate and death-rate of pneumonia in the inoculated." "Where in comparative statistics we find that the difference between the inoculated and the uninoculated is after a certain time effaced, this does not necessarily indicate that the immunity of the inoculated is diminishing. We may be witnessing, instead of a descent of the level of the inoculated to the level of the uninoculated an ascent of the uninoculated to a level of the inoculated." "We recommend that prophylactic inoculation should, except only in the case where a mass-experiment is being undertaken, be applied as a routine measure to every native on recruitment." [65,66]

The results of several of these trials were subjected to critical statistical analysis by Maynard in Memoir No. 1 of the South African Institute for Medical Research,[39] which was founded in 1912 with a gift from the Witwatersrand Native Labour Association on land provided by the South African Government. On the basis of his analysis, Maynard, statistician of the Institute,[48] concluded that the attack rate of pneumonia was lessened in the first four months following inoculation but that vaccination had no significant effect on the case fatality rate. The conclusions are not surprising when one considers that the number of pneumococcal types in the vaccine was unknown and may have been quite limited and that the doses of vaccine employed were, in the light of later knowledge,[31] marginal at best.

At the time the initial trials of pneumococcal vaccine were in progress, an alternative approach to the problem of pneumonia was initiated by Samuel Evans, Chairman of the Crown Mines Company in Johannesburg. He had read Osler's essay, "Man's Redemption of Man," delivered in Edinburgh in 1910 on the death of Robert Koch[55] and describing the success of Gorgas in ridding the Panama Canal Zone of disease. Evans concluded that here was the man who might solve the health problems of the mines; and, being an individual of action, he went to visit Gorgas in the Canal Zone, where he spent several weeks in 1912 in daily contact with the sanitarian, reviewing the accomplishments that had made possible the building of the canal.[11,21] In the early days of its construction, pneumonia had been a major problem. In 1907, Gorgas wrote: "For the last sixteen months pneumonia has been very fatal among our negro laborers, being confined almost entirely to this class of labor. It affects whites very seldom. The disease seems to be in the decline now, and I look on it as epidemic in character, a good deal as it occurs in New York and Chicago. We are endeavoring to meet this by making the general sanitary conditions better with regard to food, clothing and so forth." [22] Gorgas came clearly to recognize that the incidence of pneumonia was greatest in the early months of employment and fell steadily with the implied development of immunity. In the Zone, Blacks imported from the West Indies were housed in crowded barracks. By dispersing the majority of men from barracks to huts, the problem of pneumonia was greatly alleviated, the death rate falling from 18.74 per 1000 per annum in 1906 to 1.66 in 1910. Evans succeeded in having the Transvaal Chamber of Mines invite Gorgas to South Africa; and, after a visit to England during which he lunched with Sir Almroth Wright, Gorgas sailed for Cape Town with his wife, Major R. E. Noble and Samuel T. Darling, the first to describe histoplasmosis.[21]

Two more contrasting personalities than Gorgas and Wright could scarcely be found. Gorgas was born in 1854 in Alabama. His father, head of the University of the South at Sewanee, had been a general and Chief Ordinance Officer of the Confederate Army; and the family suffered considerable hardship at the end of the War between the States. It was young Gorgas' dream to go to West Point, but his appointment failed; and he elected a career in medicine as an alternate route to joining the army through its medical department. He graduated from Bellevue Medical College in New York in 1879 and enlisted in the military immediately thereafter. In 1882, while at Fort Brown, Texas, he survived an attack of yellow fever, an event which made him the only medical officer in the army other than Surgeon-General Sternberg immune to yellow fever at the outbreak of the Spanish-American War.[43] He is described in his anonymously written memorial in the Transactions of this Association, to which he was elected to honorary membership in 1916, as "a man of an unusually kindly and affable disposition . . . with . . . other qualities which contributed largely to the completeness of his achievements—great tenacity of purpose and endless patience." Unlike Wright, he did not engage in polemics. His modus operandi was "to find reasonable means for meeting reasonable objections."[43] As noted in the memorial cited: "It was perhaps fortunate that General Gorgas was not a laboratory man or a research worker devoted to the intense cultivation of narrow fields, but by taste a medical practitioner and by training a sanitarian who had handled broad problems and had a wide view of medicine."

Gorgas and his party arrived in Johannesburg in December, 1913, for a stay of just under three months. After a careful study of the mine labor force, he made a number of recommendations to the industry including dispersal of the miners from barracks into huts, establishment of a central hospital facility for the mines staffed by full time rather than by part time medical officers, and a change in the dietary regimen. He advised also that the Chamber of Mines appoint a chief sanitarian, answerable only to the Chamber rather than to the individual mines, to establish standards for the industry.[23] Gorgas recognized the potential value of vaccination. "It would be useful for the Chamber of Mines," he wrote, "to continue the experimental inoculation against pneumonia, using different strains of pneumococci. If we had such a vaccine, . . . then the question of the employment of the tropical natives would be at once solved. I recommend that in the future when vaccinating natives, one-half be kept as controls."[23]

Gorgas' report was received not without criticism from the local profession. In an editorial in the Medical Record of South Africa of April 14, 1914, the following appeared: "The medical reader conversant with the history of these matters on the Reef will notice that there is nothing new in any of these proposals; all these proposals have been discussed over and over again by mine medical officers and others interested in these problems. But, unfortunately, no new facts are arrayed in support of the proposals, while some of the reasons urged for their adoption are, it seems to us, based on a lack of appreciation of local conditions." The editorial concluded that acceptance of the report might result in promises made but unfulfilled, in the expenditure of thousands of pounds which might better be spent for health and in damage to the credibility of medical science for acting without further investigation.[18]

By the end of 1914, therefore, two honorary members of this Association had visited South Africa in an effort to solve the pressing problem of pneumonia in the gold mining industry; and each was to leave a protégé to carry on his work. The seriousness of the issue was highlighted when, in April, 1913, the government of South Africa forbade the further importation of so-called Tropicals, men from north of latitude 22° South, to work in the mines because of their high mortality from pneumonia.

The man who took up the work of Sir Almroth Wright was F. Spencer Lister. Lister was born in Nottinghamshire, England, in 1875. After qualifying as a physician, he worked a short time as the doctor on a cable-laying ship, arriving in South Africa in 1907. Following a brief period of private practice in Natal, he became a medical officer, first at the Premier Diamond Mine near Pretoria, and then at the Bantjes Gold Mine on the Reef, where he developed an interest in pneumonia. In 1911, he joined Sir Almroth Wright as an assistant in the first trials of pneumococcal vaccines.[20,47]

Lister was struck by the infrequency with which recently isolated pneumococci were opsonized by the sera of pneumonic patients, although occasionally the phenomenon was observed. He hypothesized that, if one examined the serum of a patient, taken at the time of crisis, with the patient's own pneumococcus isolated by lung puncture or from blood, one might obtain the reaction more readily. Lister proceeded to test his hypothesis and found that the sera of 18 of 20 patients who recovered agglutinated and opsonized the pneumococci isolated from their respective lungs, whereas of the sera of 6 cases terminating fatally, only two reacted in this fashion. When the sera of the 20 cases were examined with the pneumococci of other patients, it quickly became evident that the organisms were serologically heterogeneous. Lister was able to classify his pneumococcal strains into four groups: A, B, C and D, of which the first two were the more common. His work was published on December 22, 1913,[30] the same year that Dochez and Gillespie, working in this country, had described independently on September 6, pneumococcal Groups I, II and III,[16] which report is recognized in a postscript to Lister's paper.

In July, 1914, Maynard initiated "Pneumonia inoculation experiment no. III."[42] Noting that Wright's vaccines prepared in South Africa contained numerous local strains the diversity of which had not been ascertained, Maynard used a vaccine which took cognizance of the several pneumococcal types identified by Lister. Although the composition and dosage of the vaccine are not included in Maynard's report, Orenstein, in a paper published in 1931,[54] states that the vaccinees received a vaccine containing a total of two billion organisms of five specific types. The experiment involved 55,900 natives, half of whom were vaccinated and half of whom served as controls. Over a ten month period, there was a 20 per cent reduction in clinically diagnosed pneumonia in the vaccinees as contrasted with the controls, a reduction comparable to that which might be expected, in the light of more recent experience,[4] to result from the use of a pentavalent vaccine. The outcome is highly statistically significant ($p < 0.0002$); and, in many ways, this experiment constitutes the best evidence obtained in any of the early South African trials of the efficacy of pneumococcal vaccine. One may surmise that, had bacteriologic studies been done demonstrating that the overall reduction of pneumonia in vaccinees was due largely to the elimination of illness caused by types in the vaccine, its prophylactic value would have been established unequivocally. None was reported, however.

Meanwhile, Lister continued his studies of immunity to pneumococcus in laboratory animals and in man. By 1916, he had identified 8 capsular types of pneumococci among 96 isolates from lung punctures of blood, had shown the development of opsonins and agglutinins both in the rabbit and in man following inoculation of monovalent and polyvalent vaccines of whole pneumococcal cells and had demonstrated the relative nontoxicity of dead pneumococci by injecting as many as forty billion intravenously in a single dose into man. He cited Wright's conclusions that: "our opsonic measurements failed to tell us (a) what is the optimum dose of pneumococcal vaccine for general use in prophylaxis. . . . (c) whether one inoculation ought to be followed up by another and if so, how soon. . . . or (f) intravenous inoculations give the best immunizing response."[31] In demonstrating that "larger doses than 1,000 millions, even of a single strain of Pneumococcus, are necessary in order to give rise to demonstrable antibodies in a Native's or European's serum," Lister made the following comment: "It would ill become me to criticize the conclusions of such a great authority as Sir Almroth Wright were I not very sure of my ground, and were I not also convinced of the necessity of attempting to overtake and correct the erroneous impressions which must have been formed in the minds of many after perusal of his Report. I am particularly indebted to Sir Almroth Wright for personal instruction in his special and ingenious methods of technique; I have used them throughout this work, and for them and their originator I have the greatest admiration." Thirty years later, Heidelberger and his associates were to show that ten billion pneumococci of types 1 or 2 yielded approximately 30 to 40 micrograms of capsular polysaccharide respectively,[27] amounts of a magnitude comparable to the 50 microgram doses of individual polysaccharides used in contemporary vaccines. In retrospect, it is clear that the doses of vaccine employed in Wright's trials had been either too small or of marginal immunogenicity at best.

On the basis of the foregoing studies, Lister undertook trials with tri- or tetravalent vaccines composed of pneumococcal groups A, B, C and, in some instances, H. The first three groups corresponded, respectively, to types 5, 1 and 2 in the American nomenclature and together had accounted for 68.9 per cent of 148 isolates typed in the preceeding five years. Bacteriologic studies were to be done on all cases.[32] In structuring his trials, Lister cited a comment made in his report of the preceeding year, derived perhaps from a statement of Wright,[65,66] which was to have a crucial impact on subsequent evaluations of the efficacy of pneumococcal vaccines and was to give rise to continuous controversy over the next two decades. In 1916, he wrote: "In the system hitherto employed on the Rand for assaying the results of prophylactic inoculation against the Pneumococcus, a certain advantage conferred upon the uninoculated has, I think, been overlooked. If Pneumonia is spread, as I believe it to be, either directly from case to case or through the agency of carriers it follows that the inoculation of half of the inhabitants of a Native compound may interrupt the chain, not only of actual pneumonic patients, but also of carriers; if the inoculation achieves this it is obvious that the uninoculated half of the population will achieve an advantage which is not allowed for in the calculations."[31] The correctness of this view, established by Colin MacLeod, another Climatologist between the years 1958 and 1971, and his associates in 1945,[37] left Lister with two options. In view of the high attack rate of pneumonia in the mine compounds, he could have elected to reduce the proportion of vaccinees in the population to a third or a quarter of the total. Alternatively, he could have elected to vaccinate the entire population of one compound and to use that of another compound as a control for comparison. Lister chose the latter course, which choice, in the light of the fluctuating rates of pneumonia in different compounds from year to year,[41] raised questions in the subsequent assessment of the vaccine's efficacy. In his controversy with Orenstein, which extended over the next two decades, he cited the statement set forth above in almost every report published on the subject.[31,32,34,36] The most convincing evidence of the efficacy of Lister's vaccine is to be found in the Crown Mines experiment.[32] Among 82 consecutive cases of lobar pneumonia investigated bacteriologically, there was not a single one associated with the three pneumococcal types in the vaccine, whereas, in the absence of controls, Lister calculated by extrapolation from other epidemiologic data that there should have been 120 had the vaccine not been employed. In his extensive review and evaluation of the early South African vaccine trials, Heffron points out how little bacteriologic work seems to have been done. He estimates that cultures were obtained from only 1 per cent of the participants who developed pneumonia in the several trials.[26]

The principal skeptic regarding the prophylactic value of pneumococcal vaccines was Alexander Jeremiah Orenstein. According to a former Phila- delphia acquaintance of his, Orenstein was born in Russia and came to the United States as a child. After graduating from Jefferson Medical College in 1905, he joined the armed forces and was sent to the Canal Zone to serve with Gorgas as one of his two senior medical officers. During Evans' visit to the Zone in 1912, Orenstein had been his guide. Although the Chamber of Mines did not accept Gorgas' recommendation to establish the post of a chief sani- tarian for the mining industry, Sir Evelyn Wallers of Central Mining—Rand Mines Ltd. elected to follow it and wrote to Gorgas asking for the name of someone who might fill the post for the Corner House group of companies.[11] Gorgas suggested Orenstein, who at that moment was in German East Africa (now Tanzania) on a mission for the German government. Orenstein accepted and came to Johannesburg with the title of Superintendent of Sanitation for Rand Mines Ltd., responsible only to the chairman of the company. This ar- rangement gave him the necessary authority to carry out much needed re- forms. Although World War I had already begun, Orenstein had to go to En- gland to qualify as a physician in South Africa. Later in the conflict, he joined the South African forces and renounced his American citizenship, remaining a citizen of South Africa until his death in 1972 at the age of 93.[12] Orenstein's incisive reports did much to improve the lot of the miner's health. He brought about reconstruction of the hospital wards and operating rooms, the introduc- tion of full time mine medical officers and the first full time radiologist, im- provement of nursing services, revision of patients' diets, the introduction of water-borne sewerage on all mines and revision of the miners' housing. The example set by Rand Mines made their practices standards which were soon adopted by the remainder of the industry. In his report to the company chair- man for 1917 he wrote: "It is very gratifying to note that the mortality from pneumonia is so steadily decreasing. From 12 per 1000 for the mines of this group in 1911 it has steadily fallen to 2.65 per 1000 in the present year. The lowest previous mortality was 4.1 per 1000 in 1914."[11]

In 1918, as a result of Lister's studies, a decision was made to inoculate all new recruits to the mines with an octavalent vaccine of whole pneumococcal cells of Lister's groups A, B, C, E, G, H, J, and K.[34] Six years later Lister, who had been knighted in 1920 for his work on the immunology of pneu- mococcus, reviewed the status of pneumonia on the mines at a meeting of the Transvaal Mine Medical Officers' Association, founded in 1921. He cited both the decline in mortality from pneumonia and the infrequency of infections caused by the epidemic groups A, B and C, attributing these changes to the wide use of the vaccine, a half to three-quarters of a million doses of which were being dispensed to the industry annually: "A good deal has been made of general hygiene as the chief factor in the decrease in pneumonia mortality," stated Lister. "Every credit must be given to the great progress made in this direction on the mines but when one reflects upon the incidence of tuberculosis, meningitis and enteric fever, this factor appears to apply to pneumonia only, which detracts somewhat from the claim put forward."[34]

The discussion of Lister's presentation was lengthy and lively and engaged in by a number of participants, some supportive, some critical, including Orenstein, who chaired the meeting. The issue of controls was raised again, and Lister quoted his view on this subject published originally in 1916. Additional topics that were discussed included the interpretation of data on morbidity and mortality as related to the use of vaccine and the possible change in the etiology and pathology of the pneumonia observed. Orenstein closed the meeting with the following remarks: "He would also like to correct a misapprehension under which Sir Spencer Lister was labouring—that he (the Chairman) had inferred that general sanitation was the deciding factor in the reduction of pneumonia incidence. All he (the speaker) had said was that pneumococcal vaccine was not the deciding factor. Most people tried to pin down improvement in morbidity and mortality, whether it be in the mortality of children, or mortality from any one disease, to one factor.

"That was a wrong mental attitude. Many factors are at work to bring about these phenomena. More particularly must this be this case in so protean a disease as pneumonia. He was convinced that vaccination was not a panacea for pneumonia."[34]

An impasse had thus been reached which could be resolved only by a suitably structured trial of the vaccine which would include adequate control subjects and bacteriologic study of all respiratory illness. In the late 1920's, there appeared to some observers, at least, to be a change in the character of pneumonia from the lobar anatomic pattern to that of bronchopneumonia,[35,59] associated perhaps with influenza viral infection although this hypothesis cannot be proved. In this period, morbidity from pneumonia rose and the use of Lister's vaccine was abandoned by some mines. Orenstein discussed the subject again in 1931 and concluded once more the evidence supporting the efficacy of pneumococcal vaccine was lacking.[54] The same year, Ordman[49] reviewed the history of pneumonia on the Witwatersrand and attributed the fall in the mortality rate from pneumonia from 12 per 1000 per annum in 1907 to 3.36 per 1000 per annum in 1929 to improved housing and the use of vaccine. He described also a change in the bacterial flora of pneumonia in the late

1920's marked by the isolation of pneumococcal types not in the vaccine and of *Streptococcus pyogenes* as well as a variety of other bacteria including *Staphylococcus aureus* and *B. influenzae*. This change in bacterial flora was accompanied by an apparent diminution of the efficacy of the pneumococcal vaccine then employed, and Ordman recommended the preparation of a "community autogenous vaccine," tailored to contain the prevalent pneumococcal types plus the other bacterial species prevailing in each mining community.

In 1935, Lister, in an extensive monograph with Ordman, reviewed once more the history and status of pneumococcal vaccines in South Africa.[36] It was to be Lister's final communication on the subject. His sudden death in 1939 while Director of the South African Institute for Medical Research deprived that country of its most distinguished medical scientist. In that report, the authors cite Gorgas' views on pneumococcal vaccine[23] but continue to adhere to Lister's beliefs about the disadvantage of including vaccinees and control subjects in a single population. Additional bacteriologic data are reported indicating a somewhat diminished role of pneumococcal groups B and C, and earlier data on the increasing role of *Streptococcus pyogenes* are cited. Attention is drawn to the similarity of the bacteriologic findings which prevailed during the influenza epidemic of 1918.[59] Two additional papers accompany Lister and Ordman's report. In the first, the impact of a vaccine containing eight types of pneumococci, streptococci, staphylococci, *Micrococcus catarrhalis* and influenza and Friedländer's bacilli on pneumonia at the Randfontein Estates Mine is described by Peall.[57] Vaccination of all new recruits was begun in 1930. From 1929, when the morbidity and mortality rates per 1000 per annum were respectively 54.02 and 8.3, these rates fell to 9.85 and 1.1 in 1933. These declines were much more striking when contrasted with the rates for all other gold mines and were interpreted as being indicative of the vaccine's efficacy. Ordman reported analogous results from the application of a community autogenous vaccine at the Roan Antelope Copper Mine in Northern Rhodesia.[50] The interpretation of this latter experiment is clouded somewhat by the reduction in deaths from all disease even though those from pneumonia showed a more marked decline.

The advent of antimicrobial therapy brought the controversy over pneumococcal vaccine, in the main, to a close. Because of the continuing high incidence of pneumonia in the mines, accentuated by removal of the ban on the importation of Tropical labor in 1935, a controlled trial of the efficacy of sulfapyridine was carried out in 1938 revealing the utility of that drug.[1] In the same period, Ordman[52] published a reconciliation of Lister's nomenclature of pneumococcal types with that set forth by Cooper and her associates[14] in the United States. The loss of six of Lister's groups and of antisera to them, however, precluded their identification. Lister's groups T and V, infections with which were limited almost entirely to miners, had no counterparts then in the American classification. Group T was identified as American type 72 in 1944 by Eddy.[17] During one of my trips to Johannesburg, I located a small amount of antiserum to group V prepared by Dr. Ordman many years earlier. Tests with this antiserum against a variety of pneumococcal strains identified it as American type 73. Both types 72 and 73 remain important causes of pneumonia and bacteremia in African Blacks although they are very rarely isolated in this country.[4]

As was true in most parts of the world, concern over pneumonia waned after the introduction first of sulfonamides and later of penicillin and of other antibiotics. Ordman's interest remained, however, and he continued to point out the high attack rate of pneumonia in Tropical miners, citing a figure of 135 per 1000 per annum in 1946. With regard to bacteriologic study of pneumonia, he pointed out that: "the efficacy of the sulfonamide drugs was so great that the clinician had no particular interest in the flora associated etiologically with his cases of pneumonia."[53] Although typing of pneumococci was continued for a time and modifications of Lister's vaccine were still administered at some mines, pneumonia appeared to have had a lesser claim on the interest of mine medical officers. It did not disappear entirely, however; for the subject was discussed in 1949 and again in 1959 at meetings of the Mine Medical Officers' Association.[58]

My involvement with the problem of pneumonia in South Africa was one of those chance happenings. As a result of studies conducted in New York between 1952 and 1962, it had become apparent that endemic pneumonia was still prevalent in the United States and that, even with penicillin therapy, the mortality rate from bacteremic infection, which exceeded 25 per cent in those over 50 years of age and in those with a variety of chronic illnesses, was unacceptably high.[6] In the absence of knowledge of the physiologic derangements that accompany pneumococcal infection and of the means to correct them, prophylaxis appeared to offer the only alternative to those at significant risk of a fatal outcome of such infection. To that end, a program was initiated in 1967 under the sponsorship of the National Institute of Allergy and Infectious Diseases to bring about the relicensure of polyvalent vaccines of pneumococcal capsular polysaccharides, which had been shown twenty-two years earlier by MacLeod and his associates to be safe and effective.[37] In 1970, at a time when we were looking for populations in which to test the efficacy of the contemporary vaccines, Sir Charles Stuart-Harris of Sheffield University in England was visiting Philadelphia and told of his trip to South Africa in 1966 to discuss respiratory disease on the mines.[11] There was still much pneumonia among the miners, he reported. At that time, Professor James H. S. Gear, Director of the South African Institute for Medical Research and Sir Spencer

Lister's son-in-law, was on sabbatical at Harvard University. Through his good offices, I was put in touch with the chief medical officers of three of South Africa's largest gold mining companies; and, as a result of these contacts, a trip was made to Johannesburg in September, 1970, to determine the feasibility of conducting vaccine trials at the mines.

The initial outcome of that visit was the establishment of bacteriologic surveillance of pneumonia at several mines through the cooperation of the Mine Medical Officers' Association, the South African Institute for Medical Research and the Chamber of Mines of South Africa. With the reinstitution of capsular typing at the Institute, it became quickly apparent that pneumococcal pneumonia, though infrequently fatal, was still rife, subsequent data demonstrating an attack rate of approximately 100 per 1000 per annum among African males coming to work for the first time on the mines. The surveillance was not without its hazards, however, as indicated by a report from the Institute shown in the figure below.

The first trial of a pneumococcal vaccine was initiated in 1972 at the East Rand Preparatory Mine in Boksburg, 15 miles east of Johannesburg. The E.R.P.M. is one of the oldest and deepest mines on the Reef, having been established in 1893. It is an unforgettable experience to descend to the deepest workings of the mine two miles below the earth's surface and a mile below sea level where rock temperatures are 125°F. The mine's labor force, derived largely from Malawi (formerly Nyassa) and Mozambique, varied during the four and a half years of the trials from 6450 to 14,100 men, who were housed in barracks in four compounds. Participation was limited to men coming to work for the first time at any mine, but no miner was required to take part and a small number declined to do so. Pneumonia is not a new problem at this mine, an epidemic there having been well described by Ordman in 1937.[51]

When MacLeod and his associates carried out their trial of a tetravalent vaccine in a military population during World War II, they demonstrated in an elegantly designed experiment the correctness of Lister's view that, when half the population was immunized, the controls derived some benefit therefrom.[37] Because of this clear demonstration, the armed forces, when testing the efficacy of meningococcal vaccine in the late 1960's and early 1970's, elected to vaccinate only 20 percent of the population at risk.[3] In the three trials of pneumococcal vaccine conducted at the E.R.P.M. which involved 12,000 miners, the studies were designed to have one third of the participants receive pneumococcal vaccine, one third meningococcal vaccine and one third a saline placebo. It was possible by this partitioning of vaccinees and of controls to demonstrate unequivocally the efficacy of both vaccines in each of the trials.

Time does not permit a detailed review of the data accumulated in these

Pneumococcal Surveillance—E.R.P.M.

No. of Investigation: 147 Pneumococcal Types	No. of Isolation: 106 Number
1	35
2	22
3	4
4	5
5	1
7	5
8	6
9	2
10	1
11	2
12	5
18	3
20	1
22	1
25	7
40	2
45	2
47	1
Untypable	1

How Isolated	Positive Blood Cultures: 15	
	Types	No.
Culture and Mouse: 77	1	9
Culture only: 77	2	1
(3 mice eaten by cat)	4	1
Mouse only: 11	8	2
	45	2

studies, some of which have been published elsewhere.[7] In summary it can be said that a vaccine containing the capsular polysaccharides of 13 different pneumococcal types in a dose of 50 μg each was 80 percent effective in preventing radiologically confirmed putative pneumococcal pneumonia and pneumococcal bacteremia and that the efficacy of seven individual components of the vaccine was established, all at a high level of statistical significance. Of additional interest was the fact that pneumococcal types 72 and 73, Lister's groups T and V, were still prevalent in these populations. Another finding of note was the occurrence in these highly susceptible men of a syndrome of pneumococcal bacteremia without apparent pneumonia, an illness in infants well known to pediatricians[9] but one not having been described heretofore in adults, so far as I am aware. These studies have established beyond question the correctness of Sir Spencer Lister's views concerning both the dose and efficacy of pneumococcal vaccines. Had it not been for his decision to structure his trials of the vaccines without the inclusion of suitable controls, the need to carry out the contemporary studies might never have arisen. This latter fact notwithstanding, much credit is his due for his pioneering studies. At this juncture, one can only surmise how much Lister may have been influenced in his decisions by his contacts with Sir Almroth Wright, whose antipathy to statistical methods has been discussed earlier.

It is one of the ironies of medical history that, in the past six months, the occurrence of pneumococci highly resistant to multiple antimicrobial agents should have been recognized for the first time in South Africa.[2] The spread of these strains, insusceptible to penicillins, cephalosporins, tetracyclines, chloramphenicol, erythromycin, clindamycin, cotrimoxazole and aminoglycosides, poses a potential problem to world health of significant proportions. In the absence of new and effective antipneumococcal drugs or of an effective prophylactic vaccine, physicians might be confronted with the alternative of returning to the treatment of pneumococcal infection with type-specific antiserum. Since the first trials of pneumococcal vaccine in the South African gold mines in 1911, therefore, we have come the full circle. In the final analysis, an ounce of prevention may indeed be worth a pound of cure.

References

1. Agranat, A. L., Dreosti, A. O., and Ordman, D.: Treatment of pneumonia with 2-(p-aminobenzenesulphonamido) pyridine (M & B 693). *Lancet* 1: 309–317, 380–384, 1939.

2. Appelbaum, P. C., Koornhof, H. J., Jacobs, M., Robins-Brown, R., Isaacson, M., Gilliland, J., and Austrian, R.: Multiple-antibiotic resistance of pneumococci—South Africa. *CDC Morb. Mort. Wkly. Rep.* 26: 285–286, 1977.

3. Artenstein, M. S., Gold, R., Zimmerly, J. G., Wyle, F. A., Schneider, H., and Harkins, C.: Prevention of meningococcal disease by Group C polysaccharide vaccine. *N. Engl. J. Med.* 282: 417–420, 1970.

4. Austrian, R.: Unpublished observations.

5. Austrian, R.: Concerning Friedländer, Gram and the etiology of lobar pneumonia, an historical note. *Trans. Am. Clin. Climat. Assn.* 71: 142–149, 1959.

6. Austrian, R., and Gold, J.: Pneumococcal bacteremia with especial reference to bacteremic pneumococcal pneumonia. *Ann. Int. Med.* 60: 759–776, 1964.

7. Austrian, R., Douglas, R. M., Schiffman, G., Coetzee, A. M., Koornhof, H. J., Hayden-Smith, S., and Reid, R. D. W.: Prevention of pneumococcal pneumonia by vaccination. *Trans. Assoc. Am. Phys.* 89: 184–192, 1976.

8. Blakesley, T. H.: A Handbook to the Microscope. The Principles of Microscopy; a Handbook to the Microscope. By Sir A. E. Wright. *Nature* 75: 386–387, 1907.

9. Bratton, L., Teele, D. W., and Klein, J. O.: Outcome of unsuspected pneumococcemia in children not initially admitted to the hospital. *J. Pediat.* 90: 703–706, 1977.

10. Brodie, W. H., Rogers, W. G., and Hamilton, E. T. E.: A contribution to the pathology of infection by the pneumococcus. *S. Afr. Med. J. (Cape Town)* 6: 258–264, 1899.

11. Cartwright, J. P.: Doctors of the Mines. Purnell, Cape Town, S. Afr., 1971.

12. Coetzee, A. M.: Alexander Jeremiah Orenstein. *S. Afr. Med. J.* 46: 1188–1189, 1972.

13. Colebrook, L.: Almroth Wright, Provocative Doctor and Thinker. Wm. Heineman-Medical Books, Ltd., London, 1954.

14. Cooper, G. M., Rosenstein, C., Walter, A., and Peizer, L.: The further separation of types among the pneumococci hitherto included in Group IV and the development of therapeutic antisera for these types. *J. Exp. Med.* 55: 531–554, 1932.

15. Cope, Z.: Almroth Wright, Founder of Modern Vaccine Therapy. Thos. Nelson & Sons, Ltd., London, 1966.

16. Dochez, A. R., and Gillespie, L. J.: A biologic classification of pneumococci by means of immunity reactions. *J.A.M.A.* 61: 727–730, 1913.

17. Eddy, B. E.: Nomenclature of pneumococcic types. *U.S. Pub. Health Rep.* 59: 449–451, 1944.

18. Editorial: General Gorgas' Report. *Med. J. S. Afr.* 9: 193–195, 1914.

19. Editorial: Sir Almroth Wright's Lecture. *S. Afr. Med. Rec.* 10: 77–78, 1912.

20. Gear, J. H. S.: Personal communication.

21. Gorgas, M. D., and Hendrick, B. J.: William Crawford Gorgas, His Life and His Work. Lea & Febiger, Philadelphia, 1924.

22. Gorgas, W. C.: Sanitation in the Canal Zone. *J.A.M.A.* 46: 6–8, 1907.

23. Gorgas, W. C.: Recommendation as to sanitation concerning employees of the mines on the Rand made to the Transvaal Chamber of Mines. *J.A.M.A.* 62: 1855–1865, 1914.

24. Greenwood, M.: On methods of research available in the study of medical problems with special reference to Sir Almroth Wright's recent utterances. *Lancet* 1: 158–165, 1913.

25. Greenwood, M.: Obituary: Almroth Edward Wright. *Lancet* 1: 656, 1947.

26. Heffron, R.: Lobar Pneumonia with Special Reference to Pneumococcus Lobar Pneumonia. Commonwealth Fund, New York, 1939. pp. 448–463.

27. Heidelberger, M., MacLeod, C. M., Kaiser, S. J., and Robinson, B.: Antibody formation in volunteers following injection of pneumococci or their type-specific polysaccharides. *J. Exp. Med.* 83: 303–320, 1946.

28. J. K. M.: Transactions of the American Climatological Association for 1898. *S. Afr. Med. J.* 7: 161–162, 1899.

29. Letcher, O.: The Gold Mines of Southern Africa. Arno Press. New York, 1974. pp. 78–82.

30. Lister, F. S.: Specific serological reactions with pneumococci from different sources. *Pub. S. Afr. Inst. Med. Res.* 2: 103–116, 1913.

31. Lister, F. S.: An experimental study of prophylactic inoculation against pneumococcal infection in the rabbit and in man. *Pub. S. Afr. Inst. Med. Res.* 8: 231–287, 1916.

32. Lister, F. S.: Prophylactic inoculation of man against pneumococcal infections, and more particularly against lobar pneumonia. *Pub. S. Afr. Inst. Med. Res.* 10: 304–322, 1917.

33. Lister, F. S., and Taylor, E.: Observations and experimental investigations in epidemic influenza. *Pub. S. Afr. Inst. Med. Res. Mem. No.* 12: 1–23, 1919.

34. Lister, S.: The use of pneumococcal vaccine. *S. Afr. Med. Rec.* 22: 115–122, 138–149, 162–166, 1924.

35. Lister, S.: A note on the aetiology of epidemic influenza and secondary pneumonia. *J. Med. Assoc. S. Afr.* 5: 179–181, 1929.

36. Lister, S., and Ordman, D.: The epidemiology of pneumonia on the Witwatersrand goldfields and the prevention of pneumonia and other allied acute respiratory diseases in native labourers in South Africa by means of vaccine. *Pub. S. Afr. Inst. Med. Res.* 7: 1–81, 1935.

37. MacLeod, C. M., Hodges, R. G., Heidelberger, M., and Bernhard, W. G.: Prevention of pneumococcal pneumonia by immunization with specific capsular polysaccharides. *J. Exp. Med.* 82: 445–465, 1945.

38. Maynard, G. D.: The economic aspect of preventable deaths; being an enquiry into the financial loss due to unnecessary mortality in the Transvaal. *Tvl. Med. J.* 3: 162–168, 1908.

39. Maynard, G. D.: An enquiry into the etiology, manifestations and prevention of pneumonia amongst natives on the Rand recruited from Tropical areas. *Pub. S. Afr. Inst. Med. Res.* 1: 1–101, 1913.

40. Maynard, G. D.: Memorandum of Rand Mines pneumococcic vaccine experiment. *Med. J. S. Afr.* 9: 91–95, 1913.

41. Maynard, G. D.: Interim report of work undertaken in connection with pneumonia amongst natives in tropical areas. *Med. J. S. Afr.* 9: 208–211, 1914.

42. Maynard, G. D.: Pneumonia inoculation experiment no. III. *Med. J. S. Afr.* 11: 36–38, 1915.

43. Memorial: General William Crawford Gorgas. *Trans. Am. Climat. Clin. Assn.* 37: xxi–xxv, 1921.

44. Morgenroth, J., and Levy, R.: Chemotherapie der Pneumokokkeninfection. *Klin. Wochenschr.* 48: 1560–1561, 1979–1983, 1911.

45. Nathan, E. A.: A report on pneumonia at the Premier Diamond Mine. *Tvl. Med. J.* 2: 154–159, 1907.

46. Neufeld, F., and Händel, L.: Weitere Untersuchungen über Pneumokokken-Heilsera. III. Mitteilung. Über Vorkommen und Bedeutung atypischer Varietäten der Pneumokokkus. *Arb. a. d. kaiser. Gesundhtsamte.* 34: 293–304, 1910.

47. Obituary. Sir Frederick Spencer Lister. *S. Afr. Med. J.* 13: 685–687, 1939.

48. Obituary, G. D. Maynard, O.B.E., F.R.C.S. (Edin.), M.R.C.S., L.R.C.P. *Med. J. S. Afr.* 19: 60–61, 1923.

49. Ordman, D.: Pneumonia in the native mine workers on the Witwatersrand gold-fields. *J. Med. Assoc. S. Afr.* 5: 108–116, 1931.

50. Ordman, D.: Pneumonia in the native mine labourers of the Northern Rhodesia copperfields with an account of an experiment in pneumonia prophylaxis by means of a vaccine on the Roan Antelope Mine. *Pub. S. Afr. Inst. Med. Res.* 7: 97–124, 1935.

51. Ordman, D.: An epidemic of pneumonia amongst the native labourers on a mine on the Witwatersrand goldfields. *Proc. Tvl. Mine Med. Off. Assn.* 17: 3–10, 1937.

52. Ordman, D.: Pneumococcus types in South Africa. A study of their occurrence and distribution in the population and the effect thereon of prophylactic inoculation. *Pub. S. Afr. Inst. Med. Res.* 9: 1–27, 1938.

53. Ordman, D.: The incidence and control of pneumonia in the native labourers of the Witwatersrand goldfields. *Proc. Tvl. Mine Med. Off. Assn.* 28: 75–83, 1949.

54. Orenstein, A.J.: Vaccine prophylaxis in pneumonia. *J. Med. Assoc. S. Afr.* 5: 339–346, 1931.

55. Osler, W.: Man's Redemption of Man. A Lay Sermon, McEwan Hall, Edinburgh, Sunday, July 2nd, 1910. Constable & Co. Ltd., London, 1910.

56. Pasteur, L.: (with MM. Chamberland and Roux). Sur une maladie nouvelle provoquée par la salive d'un enfant mort de la rage. *C. r. Acad. Sci. (D) (Paris)* 92: 159–165, 1881.

57. Peall, P. A.: Prophylactic inoculation against pneumonia and other acute respiratory diseases with vaccine on the Randfontein Estates Mine. *Pub. S. Afr. Inst. Med. Res.* 7: 83–95, 1935.

58. Smit, P.: Acute respiratory disease in the African. *Proc. Mine Med. Off. Assoc.* 38: 92–101, 1959.

59. South African Institute for Medical Research. Annual Report for the Year ended 31st December, 1919. Johannesburg, 1920, pp. 22–27.

60. *S. Afr. Med. J.* 7: 167, 1899.

61. Sternberg, G. M.: A fatal form of septicemia in the rabbit produced by sub-cutaneous injection of human saliva. *Nat'l Board of Health Bull.* 2: 781–783, 1881.

62. Waldron, F. W.: Epidemic pneumonia with special reference to its infectious nature in native compounds. *S. Afr. Med. Rec.* 2: 29–31, 1904.

63. Weichselbaum, A.: Ueber die Aetiologie der acuten Lungen- und Rippenfellent-zündungen. *Medizinische Jahrbücher* 1: 483–554, 1886.

64. Wright, A. E.: British Medical Association C.G.H. (Western) Branch Annual Lecture: Principles of vaccine therapy. *S. Afr. Med. Rec.* 10: 78–82, 1912.

65. Wright, A. E., Parry Morgan, W., Colebrook, L., and Dodgson, R. W.: Observations on prophylactic inoculation against pneumococcus infections, and on the results which have been achieved by it. *Lancet* 1: 1–10, 87–95, 1914.

66. Wright, A. E.: Drugs and Vaccines in Pneumonia. On Pharmaco-therapy and Preventive Inoculation Applied to Pneumonia in the African Native. Constable & Co., Ltd., London, 1914.

9

Tracking the Identity of Lister's Pneumococcal Groups T and V (Danish Types 45 and 46)

Intimations of the serologic diversity of pneumococci, isolated independently in 1880 by Sternberg and by Pasteur, began to appear shortly before the end of the nineteenth century. In June 1897, Bezançon and Griffon,[1] attempting to devise an analogue of the Widal test to be used in the diagnosis of pneumococcal infection, described the pneumococcal agglutinating capacity of sera derived from experimentally infected animals and from naturally infected humans. For their test organism, they used a strain of pneumococcus recovered in December 1896, from the heart's blood of a mouse inoculated with sputum from a man with pneumonia. In all, Bezançon and Griffon studied the sera of seven patients with pneumonia. The sera of five patients agglutinated their test strain of pneumococcus; but those of two cases, one with a necrotizing pneumonia and the other with purulent pleurisy of long duration, failed to do so. The organism recovered from the case of necrotizing pneumonia had some attributes similar to those of pneumococcus type 3. Of the two latter cases, the authors wrote: "In these two cases, the absence of the agglutinating reaction in the serum seeded with the common pneumococcus ('le pneumocoque vulgaire') permits us to see that, besides the common pneumococcus, there exist some other races of pneumococcus, which, from the point of view of agglutination, behave as different microbes." They concluded that these findings, plus the difficulty in culturing pneumococcus, made it unlikely that serodiagnosis could be applied to the diagnosis of pneumococcal infection as it is in the diagnosis of typhoid fever.

In the ensuing 13 years, additional observations suggesting the heterogeneity of pneumococcal types appeared, culminating in the report of Neufeld and Händel, which established this fact in 1910.[2] The history of this period has been reviewed both by White[3] and by Heffron.[4]

In 1911, Sir Almroth Wright, who is usually credited with the development of typhoid vaccine, went from England to South Africa to attempt to reduce by prophylactic inoculation the ravages of pneumococcal pneumonia among gold miners in that country.[5] Although Neufeld and Händel's report indicating the existence of at least two serotypes of pneumococcus had appeared the year before, there is no indication in the publications of Wright and his colleagues that cognizance was taken of this fact in the preparation of the pneumococcal vaccines employed in the initial field trials. Among Wright's associates in these investigations was F. Spencer Lister.[6]

Frederick Spencer Lister was born in Nottinghamshire, England, in 1875. He was educated in Cambridgeshire and, after attending St. Bartholomew's Hospital, qualified as M.R.C.S. in 1905. Thereafter, he served for a time as the doctor aboard a cable-laying ship and arrived in South Africa in 1907. Electing to remain in that country and following a brief period in private practice, he became associated with the mining industry. There he developed an interest in pneumonia which led to his association with Wright when the latter came to Johannesburg. It was an association that stimulated Lister's continuously productive investigations of the pneumococcus over the ensuing quarter century.

In his early studies with Wright, Lister was struck by the infrequency with which recently isolated strains of pneumococci were opsonized, even with serum of the patient from whom they were recovered. Reasoning that serum obtained at the time of crisis might opsonize the organism causing illness, Lister took isolates from blood or from material obtained by lung puncture and examined the immunologic responses in 20 cases of pneumonia meeting these criteria. Among the 14 cases which recovered, opsonization and agglutination by the patient's serum of the pneumococci causing infection were observed in 12, whereas among the six who died, these phenomena were noted only in two.[7] There are several explanations for the probable failure to detect opsonins in the blood of most patients who died. Death may have occurred sufficiently early in illness to have provided too little time for antibodies (opsonins) to have developed; they are not usually detectable in the serum until a week or more has elapsed following the onset of illness. Second, the patient may have absorbed in the course of severe illness sufficient bacterial capsular antigen to combine with all the antibody (opsonin) produced by the patient; free antibody following recovery from pneumococcal pneumonia may not be detectable in some patients for four to eight weeks after onset of illness.

When the isolates from 18 cases of pneumonia obtained from blood or direct aspirates of the lung were examined systematically with each of the reactive sera, it became quickly apparent that the organisms were serologically heterogeneous, falling into four groups which Lister designated A, B, C, and D. Lister concluded the discussion of his findings with the following remarks:

If the validity of this method of classifying pneumococci be confirmed it will have more than one useful application. The possibility of identifying the particular strains of this organism will provide a clue as to the source of infection in different cases, and will help to elucidate the role of those pneumococcal organisms which are found so commonly in the throats of healthy individuals. The prevalence of different groups of pneumococci in different circumstances—industrial, tribal, geographical etc.—will be capable of investigation. The suggestion that second attacks of pneumonia are due to invasion by another organism can be put to the test. These and many similar enquiries may be rendered feasible.

The prophylactic pneumococcal vaccine now so extensively used on these fields may, in the light of these studies become modified; it is obvious that the efficacy of such vaccine would be enhanced if use were made of the particular strain of organism to infection by which the labourers will be exposed. It may also be found advantageous to use certain definite combinations of strains. . . .

The serum therapy of pneumonia, which has not hitherto afforded notable results, may derive additional importance when it can be used in so specific a manner as the results of these investigations lead me to hope.

Lister's report coincided closely with one describing studies conducted independently at the Rockefeller Institute, and his text bears the following postscript:

Since committing the above to paper my attention has been drawn to some recent work by A. R. Dochez and L. J. Gillespie and which has appeared in the Journal of the American Medical Association for September 6th, 1913 (pages 727–730). Although these workers have adopted different methods of investigation, yet their observations seem to have led them to conclusions somewhat similar to my own.

Over the ensuing two decades the number of pneumococcal groups identified in South Africa expanded gradually from the four defined in the initial report of 1913 to seven in 1916,[8] 10 in 1917,[9] 15 or 16 in 1931,[10] and 21 in 1935,[11] all designated by capital letters. In the same period, the serotypes of pneumococci classified originally in Dochez and Gillespie's Group IV were scrutinized in a number of laboratories in North America and in Europe, culminating in the publications of Cooper and her associates, who, by 1931, had recognized 33 capsular serotypes of pneumococci.[12] It is of historical interest to note that this immunologic classification of an encapsulated organism was accomplished without utilization of the Quellung reaction, described originally by Neufeld in 1902.[13]

In 1938, David Ordman, an associate of Lister, published a report entitled: "Pneumococcus Types in South Africa. A Study of their Occurrence and Dis-

tribution in the Population and the Effect Thereon of Prophylactic Inoculation."[14] In it, there is a reconciliation of the South African and American des-
ignations of pneumococcal types. Of 30 American capsular types (types 26
and 30 were considered identical with types 6 and 15), all but those numbered
31 and 32 had been recognized in South Africa. Of the 30 designated South
African Groups (types), all but Groups T and V had their counterparts in
Cooper's classification. It should be noted that pneumococci in South African
Groups (types) D, F, G, H, J, L, and P were not available for study and that
supplies of antiserum to these groups had been exhausted, so that it was no
longer possible to determine their identities in other schemes of classification.
The table reconciling Lister's and Cooper's nomenclatures may be found in
Appendix B of Heffron's monograph.[4]

Pneumococcal Groups T and V are cited for the first time in Lister and
Ordman's publications in 1935,[11] and the incidence of infection with the former was evidently great enough to lead to its inclusion in the polyvalent whole
bacterial vaccine used for the prevention of pneumonia at that period. In
Ordman's study of 879 pneumococcal isolates from unvaccinated native Africans with pneumonia, strains of Group T ranked seventh in frequency, accounting for 1.4 percent of all isolates, and those of Group V ranked eighth,
together with types 5 and 8, each accounting for 1.1 percent of the strains
recovered. Regrettably, no data on bacteremic illness are provided. Among
170 Europeans with pneumonia, pneumococcus Group T was recovered from
one, and there were two isolates of capsular Group V.[14]

Work on the delineation of additional pneumococcal types continued in the
1940s, both in Denmark and in the United States, and included studies of un-
classified strains provided to laboratories in both countries by Ordman. In
1944, Eddy reported that pneumococci of South African capsular Group T, a
strain of which she had received from Ordman, were identical with her strain
of capsular type 72 in the American classification.[15] Six years later, Lund, in
Denmark, published a report entitled "Four New Pneumococcus Types"
among which are included Danish capsular types 45 and 46.[16] Of these types
she wrote:

From Dr. Ordman, Johannesburg, South Africa, we have received 3 pneumococcus
strains—X4803, X2368, and W5019—that all give capsular swelling in type 45
serum. . . . Type 45 appears to be of rather frequent occurrence in South Africa,
whereas it has not yet been demonstrated in Denmark.

Type 46

In 1938 Ordman reported the pneumococcus types found in South Africa. In America, these types were compared with Cooper's types (1–32). For the type designated by

Ordman as "T", no corresponding type was at that time found in the American classification given by Cooper. Subsequently, Eddy (1944) set up "T" as type 72 (group 5).

Type "T" is of rather frequent occurrence in South Africa. Ordman found it in 1.2% of 1496 pneumonia patients and in 1.0% of 693 patients with pneumococcus meningitis. Strain "T" No. 378 was kindly sent us by Dr. Ordman who states that this strain was isolated by him in 1937 from a native miner with pneumonia.

Type "T" is not identical with any of the 73 pneumococcus types hitherto known in Denmark. . . .

Lund's observations pose a curious dilemma; for, by identifying pneumococci of South African Group (type) T with Danish capsular type 46 (American type 73), she is associating pneumococci of Group T with a different capsular type than Eddy, who identified them as belonging to American type 72 (Danish type 45). Commenting on the discrepancy seven years later, Lund stated:

By cross-absorbtion *Eddy's* type 72 is found to be identical with type 45 (Lund, 1950). . . . The strains concerned of type 45 and *Eddy* 72 were all slightly virulent for mice.

Cross-absorbtion of *Eddy's* type 73 shows identity with type 46 (Lund, 1950). Either strain reacts with type 44. Type 46 is identical with Type T which was established in South Africa by *Ordman* (1938). *Eddy* is mistaken when she declares her type 72 identical with type T (*Eddy*, 1944, p. 450). Type 46 (strain "T") and *Eddy's* strain 73 are both highly virulent for mice.[17]

It is clear that there is an unreconciled disagreement between Eddy's and Lund's classification of pneumococci of South African Group (type) T in the Danish and American nomenclatures of capsular types. Interestingly, there is no mention in any of the reports cited of pneumococci of South African Group V, a serotype found with a frequency only slightly less than that of Group T.

In November 1974, in the course of the field trials of pneumococcal vaccine being conducted then in South Africa,[18] an attempt was made to locate strains of pneumococci in groups classified by Lister which had never had their correlates in the contemporary nomenclatures of capsular types established. This search was unsuccessful; but, in the repository of Dr. Ordman's biological reagents at the South African Institute for Medical Research, several sealed ampuls of pneumococcus Group V antiserum were discovered. Two ampuls were taken to the University of Pennsylvania, and the serum was tested systematically with the Quellung reaction against a variety of pneumococcal capsular types. It reacted strongly, despite the fact that it was several decades old, with strains of pneumococcus type 46 in the Danish classification, type 73 in the American scheme. This observation was compatible with Eddy's findings but not with those of Lund, who found Ordman's type T to correspond with Danish type 46.

In 1976, two of Ordman's pneumococcal strains were obtained from Dr. Eddy, who wrote as follows: "The T strain (same as my Type 72) was marked JK: the other culture (same as my type 73) was marked 108E." Strain JK is indeed a strain of type 72 in the American classification (type 45 in the Danish), and strain 108E reacts both with antiserum to capsular type 73 in the American (type 46 in the Danish) classification and with Ordman's antiserum to capsular Group V. It would appear that, somewhere in the interchange of strains among the laboratories in Africa, Europe, and North America, a strain was mislabeled; and it may never be possible to determine with certainty the identity of Lister's pneumococci in Groups T and V. It is most likely, however, that they are represented by types 45 and 46 in the contemporary Danish classification and that type 45 represents Group T and type 46 Group V.

Nearly four decades after Ordman's reconciliation of the South African nomenclature of pneumococcal groups with Cooper's classification of capsular types, pneumococci in Groups T and V, which will be referred to hereafter respectively as types 45 and 46 in the Danish nomenclature, were still prevalent in populations of Southern African gold miners. Among 575 isolates from respiratory secretions and/or blood of patients with radiologically confirmed pneumonia or bacteremia, 63 (11 percent) were type 46 and 14 (2.4 percent) were type 45. Among 189 strains isolated from blood cultures, there were 17 (9 percent) each of types 45 and 46, placing both among the five types most frequently causing bacteremia. Most of the individuals from whom these isolates were obtained were young adult African males from Mozambique or Malawi. None had received pneumococcal vaccine.

Pneumococcal types 45 and 46 are uncommon in most other parts of the world in which studies have been done, although both have been recognized in Papua-New Guinea where type 46 was responsible in one area for 29 (25 percent) of 115 bacteremic infections.[19] In the United States, there were only two isolates of type 45 and three of type 46 among 4,335 pneumococcal strains recovered from blood cultures in the past two decades.[20] Whether or not there is a genetic predisposition to infection with these two pneumococcal types in certain ethnic groups in Southern Africa and in Papua-New Guinea is unknown, although a relationship between human genotype and susceptibility to infection with certain capsulated bacteria has been suggested, but not established, by several groups of investigators.[21,22] The structure of the capsular polysaccharides of pneumococcal types 45[23] and 46[24] has each been established recently, information which may be helpful in understanding ultimately their infectivity, and both polymers have been incorporated in experimental vaccines. The work begun by Lister and his associates 70 years ago in South Africa continues to bear fruit.

Acknowledgement. The author expresses his appreciation to the South African Institute for Medical Research and to Drs. J. H. S. Gear, H. J. Koornhof, and C. H. Wyndham for their assistance in locating and making pneumococcal Group V antiserum available.

References

1. Bezançon, F., Griffon, V.: Pouvoir agglutinatif du serum dans les infections experimentales et humaines à pneumocoques (deuxième partie). Compte rendu hebdom. Séances et Mém. de la Soc. de Biologie 49: 579–581, 1897.

2. Neufeld, F., Händel, L.: Weitere Untersuchungen über Pneumokokken-Heilsera. III. Mitteilung. Über Vorkommen und Bedeutung atypischer Varietäten der Pneumokokkus. Arb. a. d. kaiser Gesundhtsamte 34: 293–304, 1910.

3. White, B.: The Biology of Pneumococcus. Cambridge, Harvard University Press, 1979, pp. 103–118.

4. Heffron, R.: Pneumonia with Special Reference to Pneumococcus Lobar Pneumonia. Cambridge, Harvard University Press, 1979, pp.22–24; p. 947.

5. Austrian, R.: Of gold and pneumococci. A history of pneumococcal vaccines in South Africa. Trans. Amer. Clin. Climat. Assoc. 89:141–161, 1977.

6. Obituary: Sir Frederick Spencer Lister. S. Afr. Med. J. 13: 685–687, 1939.

7. Lister, F. S.: Specific serological reactions with pneumococci from different sources. Pub. S. Afr. Inst. Med. Res. 1(2): 103–116, 1913.

8. Lister, F. S.: An experimental study of prophylactic inoculation against pneumococcal infection in the rabbit and in man. Pub. S. Afr. Inst. Med. Res. 1(8): 231–287, 1916.

9. Lister, F. S.: Prophylactic inoculation of man against pneumococcal infections, and more particularly against lobar pneumonia. Pub. S. Afr. Inst. Med. Res. 1(10): 304–322, 1917.

10. Ordman, D.: Pneumonia in the native mine workers on the Witwatersrand goldfields. J. Med. Assoc. S. Afr. 5: 108–116, 1931.

11. Lister, S., Ordman, D.: The epidemiology of pneumonia on the Witwatersrand goldfields and the prevention of pneumonia and other allied acute respiratory diseases in native labourers in South Africa by means of vaccine. Pub. S. Afr. Inst. Med. Res. 7: 1–81, 1935.

12. Cooper, G., Rosenstein, C., Walter, A. et al.: The further separation of types among the pneumococci hitherto included in Group IV and the development of therapeutic antisera for these types. J. Exp. Med. 55: 531–554, 1932.

13. Austrian, R.: The Quellung reaction, a neglected microbiologic technique. Mt. Sinai J. Med. 43: 699–709, 1976.

14. Ordman, D.: Pneumococcus types in South Africa. A study of their occurrence and distribution in the population and the effect thereon of prophylactic inoculation. Pub. S. Afr. Inst. Med. Res. 9: 1–27, 1938.

15. Eddy, B. E.: Nomenclature of pneumococcic types. Pub. Health. Rep. 59: 449–451, 1944.

16. Lund, E.: Four new pneumococcus types. Acta Path. Microbiol. Scand. 27: 720–725, 1950.

17. Lund, E.: The present status of the pneumococci, including three new pneumococcus types. Acta Path. Microbiol. Scand. 40: 425–435, 1957.

18. Austrian, R., Douglas, R. M., Schiffman, G., et al.: Prevention of pneumococcal pneumonia by vaccination. Trans. Assoc. Amer. Phys. 89: 184–194, 1976.

19. Riley, I. D.: Pneumonia in Papua New Guinea. Thesis for the degree of Doctor of Medicine, the University of Sydney, 1979, pp. 111–117.

20. Austrian, R.: Unpublished observations.

21. Whisnant, J. K., Rogentine, G. M., Gralnick, M. A., et al.: Host factors and antibody response to *Haemophilus influenzae* type b meningitis and epiglottitis. J. Infect. Dis. 133: 448–455, 1976.

22. Pandey, J. P., Virella, G., Loadhold, C. B., et al.: Association between immunoglobulin allotypes and immune responses to Haemophilus influenzae and meningococcus polysaccharides. Lancet i: 190–192, 1979.

23. Daoust, V., Carlo, D. J., Zeltner, J. Y., et al.: Specific capsular polysaccharide of type 45 Streptococcus pneumoniae (American type 72). Infect. Immun. 32: 1028–1033, 1981.

24. Benzing, L., Carlo, D. J., Perry, M. B.: Specific capsular polysaccharide of type 46 Streptococcus pneumoniae. Infect. Immun. 32: 1024–1027, 1981.

10

Pneumonia in the Later Years

Although I did not have the good fortune to know Dr. Willard Owen Thompson, it is clear from what I have read of his life and accomplishments that he was one of those rare men who could catalyse others to greater achievement, both individually and collectively. His contributions to this Society are signalized by the award established in his memory; and, in accepting it today, I do so for all who have collaborated in the undertakings of the past two decades to make possible the prevention of some forms of pneumonia. You honor us all by this recognition, and I thank you most warmly, not only on my behalf, but on theirs as well.

Pneumonia, as pointed out by Heffron in his magnificent, recently republished monograph,[1] has been known to man for more than two millennia; but it is only in the last two centuries that his understanding of this disorder has evolved to permit accurate diagnosis and, in some instances, effective treatment or prophylaxis. At the outset, it should be recalled that pneumonia is not a single disease but a complex of acute inflammatory disorders of the lung of diverse causes. Of the latter, one of the most important is the pneumococcus, the commonest incitant of community-acquired bacterial pneumonia.

Data on morbidity and mortality of lobar pneumonia show marked variations in each at different stages of life. Both are high in infancy, reach their nadir at the time of puberty and rise thereafter to reach their maximums in the eighth and ninth decades. For example, in Massachusetts between 1921 and 1930, the reported attack rate of lobar pneumonia per 100,000 persons among those 80 years of age and older was 3,488, 5.4 times higher than among those 10 to 14 years of age. In similar fashion, the death rate from lobar pneumonia per 100,000 persons 80 years of age and older was 4,292, 62 times higher than for those 10 to 14 years of age.[1a] These data, although not of the most recent origins, do not differ significantly in their relationships from those of more recent acquisition, and indicate quite clearly that acute infections of the lung become a problem of increasing frequency and severity as life advances. Indeed, in 1974, among those 65 years of age and older, "Influenza and Pneumonia" ranked fourth on the list of causes of death.[2] Because some illnesses in this diagnostic category may be treatable or preventable or both, they are worthy of the attention of physicians, especially those whose major concern is the care of the elderly.

Early Observations in Relation to Geriatrics

Although some look upon geriatrics as a relatively new subspeciality of medicine, interest in disease in the older segments of the population dates back, according to Charcot, to the eighteenth century. In his treatise entitled: "Lessons on the Maladies of the Aged and on Chronic Disease,"[3] published in 1868, he wrote as follows:

"And yet, gentlemen, this facet of medicine, so interesting, has long been neglected, and it is scarcely only in our time that it has succeeded in gaining its autonomy. It is an epoch very close to ours, in France, and in this very hospital, that has constituted and affirmed, in all its originality, so to speak, the pathology of the aged. Before this epoch, one could scarcely cite where the aspect of the illnesses of old age had been entertained. If one accepts the little treatise of Floyer published in 1724, the more recent work of Welsted and finally that of Fischer, published in 1776, the greater part of medical works of the past century which dealt in a special manner with the senile period had an aspect above all literary or philosphic: they are more of less ingenious paraphrases of the famous treatise *de Senectute* of the Roman orator."

The work "in this very hospital" to which Charcot referred was initiated by Pinel in 1815 and was followed by a series of five reports emanating from the Salpêtrière in Paris written by MM. Hourmann and Dechambre and published in the Archives générales de Médicine in 1835 and 1836,[4-8] less than twenty years after Laennec's classic description of pneumonia. Headed "Clinical research to serve as an account of the illnesses of the aged," the articles are subtitled "Maladies of the organs of respiration," "Respiration in the aged" and "Pneumonia in the aged," the last appearing in three parts. They are a testament to the utility of careful observation carried out before the introduction of clinical thermometry, microbiology and radiology, all indispensable tools of physicians today; and it seems worthwhile to cite some of the clinical findings of these astute investigators.

The Salpêtrière served as an asylum in the first half of the last century for approximately 2,500 women of whom the majority belonged to the less favored classes of society but among whom some had known better days. They comprised two distinct groups, one made up predominantly of those more than 70 years of age in otherwise good health who, because of misery or abandonment, had been placed under the protection of public assistance. It was this group that provided the material for the study of the affections of old age. A second group included women of all ages stricken for the most part with chronic, reputedly incurable diseases which had reduced them to a state of permanent infirmity.

Hourmann and Dechambre studied 156 patients with pneumonia: 103 died and autopsies were performed on 67 of them. Of the predisposing causes, in addition to habitual bronchorrhea and more or less marked permanent congestion of the lungs, these authors wrote: "We note under this category of first importance the rigidity of all the mechanical apparatus of respiration which impedes not only the passage of air and the expectoration of bronchial mucus but clogs also the pulmonary circulation; coming next are the organic affections of the heart and great vessels, so varied and so common in old age and the effect of which is the same, as well as the diverse abdominal swellings which compress the diaphragm and the thoracic organs, above all that which is due to distention of the intestines by gas of which the inertia of its walls permits expulsion only with difficulty." [7] Charcot's observations on pulmonary function in the aged three decades later in 1868 accord with those of these early investigators. "The respiratory functions are equally diminished in their ensemble which are manifested at once by the diminution of the quantity of carbonic acid exhaled, by augmentation of the number of inspirations and by the reduction of the vital capacity of the lungs: this last result, according to the spirometric research of Wintrich, of Schepf and of Geist, begins to manifest itself at about the age of 35 years, and reaches its maximum at 65 to 76 years." [3]

The association of pneumonia with the colder months of the year was noted in the entire series of patients and confirmed in the autopsied group. Abrupt changes in temperature were believed to be of greater importance than sustained low readings of the thermometer; and, although the observation of Hippocrates that a northeast wind predisposed to pneumonia was borne out, the period in which it prevailed was accompanied by low and variable temperatures.

Contemporary writing on infections in the aged calls attention to their frequently insidious onset and to the paucity of symptoms directing attention to the affected organ system. The following passages from Hourmann and Dechambre are telling: "Pneumonia in the aged begins in two perfectly distinct ways; at times abruptly and with the cortege of symptoms which herald it habitually in the adult; at times slowly, indistinctly, and in the absence of symptoms. . . . In the second form of onset, one observes neither chill, nor pleural pain: a general malaise, some weakness, augmentation or irregularity of respiratory movements, a little irregular cough, some warmth of the skin, here often the sole events which signal the inflammatory invasion of the lungs. But it happens often that all these symptoms are not found united. There may be at times neither warmth of the skin, cough nor disorder of respiration and all that one observes is the general malaise and weakness.

"Finally in several more obscure cases, our elderly ladies do not even complain of weakness or of malaise. They do not ask to come to the infirmary; no one in their dormitory, neither the attendants, the maids nor their neighbors sees a change in their situation. They arise, make their bed, walk about and eat as usual, then feeling a little tired, they lie down on their bed and expire. This is true of the *deaths* called *sudden*, of old age at the Salpêtrière, ... For example, a poor woman of 85 years, sleeping in bed No. 12 in the halle St. Alexandre, admitted seven days earlier because of a simple indigestion, talked to us gaily and to prove to us her good appetite, chewed with great effort a biscuit of Rheims: the visit to the hall was not finished when someone came to us to announce that the woman was dying. Arriving in great haste, we received her last sigh; her lips still retained the remains of the biscuit. On opening the body, we found the lower lobe of the right lung in full suppuration throughout its entire thickness. The larynx, trachea and bronchi were perfectly free of all foreign bodies . . ." Again: ". . . it is important to take account of insanity to appreciate all the conditions which render inflammation latent. The old woman whom it concerned, *The queen of all places*, was remarkable for her loquacity and the vigor of the intonations of her voice. One morning, without any indication of the slightest morbid change in her to the point where she promenaded and perorated with the same energy and delirium as usual one saw her fall and soon die. One entire lung had been converted to gray hepatization."[7]

In their final report, Hourmann and Dechambre make additional observations. They note that pneumonia is rare in the aged without some derangement of mental faculties—delirium fleeting or continuing, tranquil or agitated, usually worse at night and having often the character of a weakening of cerebral faculties. The frequent failure of the pulse to indicate fever and the commonness of its irregularity in this age group are also cited.

More remarkable, however, are the observations on the state of the blood in the elderly pneumonic patient at a time antedating its routine microscopic examination.[8] Noting that: "The existence of an inflammatory buffy coat is considered everywhere as an all but immutable characteristic in inflammation to the point where the name *pneumonic* buffy coat has been advanced. . . . In effect, it is only in a minority of the cases that the pneumonia (in the aged) is accompanied by the typical state of the buffy coat of the blood. Of twenty-five

bleedings taken from subjects who succumbed, it was present only eight
times. It was present nine times among 23 who were bled and followed by
recovery, in all, in 17 of 47 bleedings.

"In the 17 cases in which the inflammatory buffy coat was demonstrated,
the onset was latent in one and acute in 15. In one case, it was not determined.

"In the thirty cases where the increased buffy coat was lacking, the onset
was latent in 11 and acute in 18; again in one case it was not noted. From this
it follows that the augmented state of the buffy coat is manifested more frequently in the acute form, that is to say, in the frankly inflammatory form of
the disease." Three quarters of a century later, Chatard, reviewing cases
of acute lobar pneumonia at the Johns Hopkins Hospital was to observe:
"After 30 years the leucocytosis seems to be less marked, and this is most
apparent after 50 years; the mortality in these years with low grades of leucocytosis is high. Of twelve patients above 55 years with a leucocytosis below
15,000 per cmm, all died."[9] It should be noted, however, that data on leukocyte counts prior to the patients' becoming acutely ill are lacking for the elderly with pneumonia, and it is not clear whether the absence of leukocytosis
is the result of a state antedating infection or a reflection of the toxemia that
accompanies it.

More recent writings bear out the accuracy of many of the cited observations of the last century.[10] In a study of 2,033 sudden and unexpected natural
deaths in New York City occurring between 1937 and 1943, the cause of
which was determined by autopsy, 176 deaths, or 1 in 12, were attributed to
lobar pneumonia and an additional 133 to bronchopneumonia.[11] In a more recent study of elderly patients in England from whom blood for culture was
taken because of the onset of confusion, respiratory infection, nonspecific
malaise, loss of control of diabetes or of suspected subacute bacterial endocarditis, 7 of 27 organisms isolated proved to be pneumococci, the commonest bacterial species recovered.[12] From this limited sampling of clinical
reports, it is clear that the clinician caring for elderly patients must have a
high index of suspicion of the presence of infection and an awareness of the
atypical nature of the presentation of such illnesses as pneumonia, including
that caused by pneumococcus, in the aged.

In 1889, Townsend and Coolidge reviewed 1,000 cases of lobar pneumonia,
all that had been admitted to the Massachusetts General Hospital since the first
case in 1822.[13] This study, the results of which were confirmed by Shattuck
and Lawrence, who extended the observations at the same hospital from 1889
to 1917,[14] showed a clear and steady rise in the mortality from lobar pneumonia with increasing age, from approximately 10 percent in the second decade of life to 66 percent in the seventh decade. One of the discussants of the

earlier paper commented: "I have only one remark to make: it seems to me a most valuable paper. I want to suggest that it ought to stimulate us in every way to try to find some means of preventing—if we cannot cure it."

Age and Defense Mechanisms, with Special Reference to Pneumonia

The reasons for the increased incidence of pneumonia which accompanies the latter decades of life have not been delineated clearly. The defenses of the normal lung against bacterial invasion are multiple and efficient, and bacteria inhaled in droplets small enough to reach the pulmonary alveoli of experimental animals are usually cleared without the development of significant pulmonary lesions.[15] Only when the epithelial lining of the lower repiratory tract is altered by viral, chemical or physical injury or when pulmonary edema, local or general, develops is bacterial pneumonia likely to ensue.[16] It was recognized more than a century ago[3] and confirmed in modern times[17] that significant changes in the ventilatory apparatus take place with advancing age, changes which undoubtedly interfere with the cleansing of the respiratory tract and increase vulnerability to pulmonary infection. Aspiration of food and drink by the debilitated, especially when ingesting either in the supine position, may well be the initiating factor of pneumonia.[18]

Much attention has been given to the effect of age on the host's defensive mechanisms against infection. Although alterations with age both of humoral and of cellular functions can be demonstrated, no single factor has emerged as the one responsible for either the increased morbidity or the mortality from infection in later life.[19-21] There is a clear need to study a large cohort of subjects over a period of several decades, and to attempt to relate quantitatively a number of host defenses to the clinical history of each subject.

In contrast to general resistance of the lower respiratory tract to bacterial infection, which resistance is related to its anatomic and physiologic integrity, immunity to pneumococcal infection can be correlated significantly with the presence of circulating type-specific anticapsular antibodies. Their role is to increase the efficiency of phagocytosis of pneumococci by polymorphonuclear leukocytes which, in turn, destroy the ingested bacteria. Type-specific anticapsular antibody has no direct deleterious effect on pneumococci, either in the presence or in the absence of complement, and cannot be expected to bring about recovery from pneumococcal infection in the absence of actively functioning phagocytes.

Age-related studies of antibodies to type-specific pneumococcal capsular polysaccharides and of the bactericidal activity of whole blood against several pneumococcal types demonstrate the passive transfer of maternal antibody, if present, to the fetus. Antibody acquired in this fashion declines rapidly during the first six months of life, after which time actively acquired antibody begins to develop as a result either of direct contact with specific pneumococcal types or with bacteria possessing carbohydrate antigens cross-reacting with those of pneumococci. Levels of antibody comparable to those seen in adults are achieved in the latter part of the second decade of life.[22] Studies of the bactericidal activity of the blood of humans of different ages by Finland and Sutliff show such activity well maintained in later life against some pneumococcal types but not fully so against all.[23, 24] The significance of their findings, in clinical terms, is difficult to assess; for the amount of antibody or the titer of the bactericidal activity of the blood required to protect a person against type-specific pneumococcal infection is unknown and may differ with the immunoglobulin class of antibody and the capsular type of the infecting organism.

The desirability of preventing pneumococcal pneumonia in the aged is borne out clearly by studies of proved bacteremic pneumococcal pneumonia in patients over the age of 50 treated with penicillin or with other potent antipneumococcal drugs.[25-27] Among 160 patients of this age with bacteremic pneumococcal pneumonia uncomplicated by an extrapulmonary focus of infection and treated with penicillin, 44 or 28 percent succumbed.[25] The utility of studying bacteremic pneumococcal pneumonia relates to several issues. Bacteremia, when present, provides a definitive causal diagnosis of pneumonia and obviates the need for transtracheal or lung puncture. Such a procedure would be required, in the absence of bacteremia, to establish the role of an organism which might be carried in the upper respiratory tract of healthy subjects. In addition, bacteremia is an index of severe infection, the prognosis being about two to four times less favorable in its presence than in its absence, whether or not the patient receives specific antipneumococcal therapy.[28] There is, in addition, strongly suggestive evidence that the proportion of putative and proved pneumococcal pneumonias accompanied by bacteremia increases with age.[1b]

The adverse effect upon prognosis of complicating underlying systemic illness at any age on the outcome of bacteremic pneumococcal pneumonia treated with penicillin is attested by the comparably high fatality rate of 27 percent among 236 such patients.[25] As might be anticipated, the association of such chronic disorders as cardiac disease, pulmonary disease, hepatic or renal disease, diabetes and other endocrinopathies, blood dyscrasias and neoplasms with bacteremic pneumococcal pneumonia was higher in the elderly than in their infected younger counterparts. Those of any age with functional or anatomic asplenia were also at high risk. Mortality was especially high (49 percent) among 55 patients with cardiac disease in whom bacteremic pneumococcal pneumonia developed. The infection tended also to be insidious in onset in some patients with chronic pulmonary congestion, running a brief but lethal course not too different from that described in the last century by authors cited earlier. In fact, the diagnosis might well have been missed had it not been routine practice to obtain cultures of blood from all febrile hospitalized patients. It is impossible to overstress the importance and diagnostic value of the blood culture, obtained *before* the administration of antimicrobial drugs, in the management of the elderly patient with or without chronic underlying systemic illness. Positive results provide usually unequivocal evidence of the cause of infection and are an unequaled asset in the selection of treatment. In addition to the atypical physical findings of pneumonia in the elderly, the changes in roentgenographic studies of the chest may also be unusual, an observation highlighted by Ziskind and collaborators in an investigation of radiologic findings in bacteremic pneumococcal pneumonia.[29]

If one examines the curves of survival with time of groups of patients with bacteremic pneumococcal pneumonia treated symptomatically, or with type-specific anticapsular serum, or with penicillin, an interesting finding emerges.[25] The three curves are essentially superimposable during the first five days following the onset of illness. This observation suggests that, for patients sustaining irreversible physiologic injury very early in the course of illness, antibacterial therapy, whatever its nature, can do little to bring about their recovery despite its ability to halt further bacterial multiplication. In the absence of knowledge of the precise nature of the physiologic injury brought about by pneumococcal infection, efforts to correct the damage remain empirical and are often unsuccessful. Until a better understanding of the derangements which accompany pneumococcal infection is available, prophylaxis offers the only alternative at hand to protect those at high risk of a fatal outcome from such illness.

Prevention—Vaccines

Attempts to prevent pneumococcal pneumonia by vaccination date from 1911 when the assistance of Sir Almroth Wright, the developer of typhoid vaccine, was enlisted by the South African gold mining industry to find a means of controlling the ravages of pneumococcal disease among its workers.[30] At the time, neither the diversity of pneumococcal types nor the proper dose of bacteria required to immunize man was known, and the efficacy of the vaccines used by Wright is moot, at best. His protégé, Sir F. Spencer Lister, succeeded in solving a number of problems relating to the formulation of vaccines of intact killed pneumococci; and he might have demonstrated their efficacy had he structured more suitably his trials designed to demonstrate it. The subsequent recognition of the antigenicity of pneumococcal capsular polysaccharides in the mouse in 1927[31] and in man in 1930[32] led in later trials to the use of vaccines composed of these chemically defined antigens. A trial conducted in the early 1940's in a military population in which pneumococcal pneumonia was epidemic provided for the first time unequivocal evidence that immunization of man with pneumococcal capsular polysaccharides provided a high degree of protection against infection with the homologous pneumococcal types.[33] Although two hexavalent vaccines, shown to be safe and to stimulate antibodies persisting as long as five to eight years,[34] were made available commercially as a sequel to these studies, their appearance coincided with the introduction of several potent antipneumococcal drugs. Because a need for vaccines was not perceived at the time, they were not used and consequently were removed from the market. When it was demonstrated subsequently that there are segments of the population remaining at high risk of a fatal outcome despite the availability of potent antipneumococcal drugs, a decision to redevelop polyvalent vaccines of pneumococcal capsular polysaccharides was made.

To bring about the relicensure of a pneumococcal vaccine, the pneumococcal types most frequently causing bacteremic infection were determined, the dose of each capsular polysaccharide most suitable for immunization was ascertained, the safety of the vaccine was established and its efficacy in preventing infection in populations at risk of pneumococcal infection was investigated. Field trials of several polyvalent vaccines were conducted both in this country and abroad. Because of the continuing high attack rates of pneumococcal pneumonia in South African gold mining novices, of a magnitude of 100 or more per 1000 persons per annum, controlled trials of these vaccines, involving 12,000 young adult males, were conducted in that country. Evidence of the vaccines' 80 to 85 percent efficacy in preventing type-specific pneumococcal pneumonia and bacteremia was highly significant statistically.[35, 36]

Results derived from two trials of pneumococcal vaccine in the United States, one in a hospital for chronic disease and the other in members of a prepaid health plan all over the age of 45, are more difficult to interpret. The precise attack rate of pneumococcal pneumonia in this country is not known for a variety of reasons, but estimates based on extrapolations from existing evidence suggest that it is between 2 and 6 per 1,000 persons per annum. The attack rate of pneumococcal bacteremia is probably between 25 and 50 per 100,000 persons per annum, a rate similar to that of poliomyelitis prior to the introduction of vaccines for the prevention of that disease.[37] Populations of 200,000 or more subjects were required to demonstrate the efficacy of the vaccine to prevent poliomyelitis but were not available for comparable investigation of the ability of pneumococcal vaccine to prevent bacteremia. It was necessary, therefore, to use serologic confirmation of nonbacteremic pneumococcal infections in the smaller populations in which the vaccine was studied in the United States. Interpretation of serologic data from vaccinated persons is uncertain because re-injection of bacterial polysaccharide antigens often is followed by a very limited immunologic response, or by none. If one accepts the foregoing limitation, the results of the two trials of pneumococcal vaccine in this country are altogether in accord with those of all other trials of pneumococcal vaccines, demonstrating on the basis of seroconversion an 80 percent protective efficacy against type-specific pneumococcal infection. They are in agreement also with an earlier trial of a less complex pneumococcal vaccine conducted by Kaufman,[38] one involving 5,000 vaccinees and 5,000 control subjects 50 years of age or older. Although some questions have been raised regarding the structure of this trial, it demonstrated in the vaccinees when contrasted with the controls, a 90 percent reduction in bacteremic infection caused by the three types in the vaccine (types 1, 2, and 3).

Studies of humoral immunity in the elderly provide little evidence suggesting that it fails in later life, although there are data that levels of antibodies to some antigens decline with aging. A classic example is that of the A,B,O blood group isoantibodies.[39] Their decline notwithstanding, it is still necessary to cross-match the elderly prior to transfusion with blood. Humoral immunity to such diseases as measles clearly persists, or one would see recurrences in the aged, evidence of which is lacking from the epidemiologic data available.[40] Although the elderly respond immunologically to tetanus toxoid,[41] the fact that many of them have not received this universally recommended prophylactic has resulted in a disproportionate amount of tetanus in this segment of the population.[40] Studies of the immunologic responsiveness of the elderly to pneumococcal capsular polysaccharides are limited but demonstrate that levels of antibodies to these antigens increase following vaccination, although the magnitude of the response by some may be less than that observed in their younger counterparts.[42] Assays of IgG_2, the immunoglobulin class in which antibodies to polysaccharides commonly are found, show no diminution in their levels in nonagenarians.[43] None of the evidence available suggests that older persons should not be immunized.

Persistence of antibodies to pneumococcal capsular polysaccharides, like that following recovery from pneumococcal infection, is long-lived. Recovery from type-specific pneumococcal infection appears to confer life-long immunity to the homologous capsular type, and it is recognized that recurrent bacteremic infection with the same capsular type is a hallmark of dysgammaglobulinemia. Studies of anticapsular antibodies in vaccinees show that the time course of their decay resembles that following recovery from infection and that antibodies persist at half to a third of their peak values following immunization as long as 5 to 8 years after a single injection of vaccine. For that reason, re-injection of pneumococcal vaccine more frequently than once every 5 years is not recommended. In addition, reactions to the vaccine have been correlated with the aggregate level of antibodies to the polysaccharide antigens in it.[44] This finding is another reason for not re-administering the vaccine at frequent intervals. Although the target populations for pneumococcal and for influenza vaccines are very similar, the different epidemiology of infections caused by these microbial agents and the dissimilar properties of their vaccines make it unsuitable to combine them in a single preparation. They may be administered simultaneously, however, should circumstances warrant, provided they are injected at separate sites from separate syringes.

Although more remains to be learned about pneumococcal vaccine and its efficacy in some segments of the population at high risk from pneumococcal infection, current knowledge concerning both its safety and efficacy warrants its more extensive use. An interesting new approach to evaluation of the vaccine, based upon a modification of the standard epidemiologic formula for assessing vaccines but eliminating the requirement for knowing the sizes of the populations of vaccinated and unvaccinated persons at risk, may facilitate its further analysis through the continued study of bacteremic infections in both groups.[45] Additional investigation will be required, however, to validate fully this potentially useful method. Preliminary study suggests that pneumococcal vaccine is 60 percent effective in preventing bacteremic infections in segments of the population over 10 years of age at high risk, even when some immuno-compromised subjects incapable of an immunologic response are included among the vaccinees.

Much of the foregoing deals with the subject of pneumococcal pneumonia. Many other infectious agents may invade the lung, and it should not be inferred that the use of pneumococcal vaccine will eliminate the problem of pneumonia any more than it should be concluded that measles vaccine will eliminate all the exanthems of childhood. Each vaccine is capable, nonetheless, of decreasing significantly the burden of human illness. It should be remembered also, when assessing pneumococcal vaccine, that in reality one is examining simultaneously 14 separate vaccines and regarding a failure of any one as a failure of all! In a theoretical model based on several assumptions regarding susceptibility, responsiveness and exposure to the pneumococcal types in the vaccine, and hypothesizing 99 percent efficacy of each of its antigens, the maximal achievable efficacy of the polyvalent formulation, if a failure of one of its components is considered as a failure of all, is 0.99^{14} or 87 percent.

Implications for the Elderly

In the early editions of his landmark textbook of medicine, Sir William Osler referred to lobar pneumonia as "the special enemy of old age."[46] In the third edition, he was to characterize it also "the friend of the aged."[47] Osler's ambivalence about old age is reflected also in his valedictory address at the Johns Hopkins University in 1905, delivered when he was 55.[48] Entitled "The Fixed Period," after Anthony Trollope's novel of the same name, it suggested retirement from active life of men over 60 years of age and "their peaceful departure by chloroform" thereafter, following a year of contemplation. The address, which Cushing describes as intended to have been half humorous, evoked a storm of negative response in the national press, which evidently caught Osler by surprise and caused him some anguish.[49] Trollope's tale, published in 1882, describes the island republic of Britannula, settled by young New Zealand expatriates, which gained its independence from the British empire.[50] Among its laws was one designed for the "abolition of the miseries, weakness and *fainéant* imbecility of old age, by the prearranged ceasing to live of those who would otherwise become old." The theme must have seemed avant garde to its author as well as to others; for, interestingly, the events are set in 1980. The story contains, among other ideas, the earliest cost-benefit analysis of which I am aware. Of the aged, John Neverbend, President of Britannula, wrote as follows:

"They would be prepared for their departure, for the benefit of their country, surrounded by all the comforts of which at their time of life, they would be susceptible, in a college maintained at the public expense; and each, as he drew nearer to the happy day, would be treated with increasing honour. I myself had gone most closely into the question of expense, and had found that by the use of machinery the college could almost be made self-supporting. But we should save on an average £50 for each man and woman who had departed. When our population should have become a million, presuming that only one in fifty would have reached the desired age, the sum actually saved to the colony would amount to £1,000,000 a-year. It would keep us out of debt, make for us our railways, render all our rivers navigable, construct our bridges and leave us shortly the richest people on God's earth! And this would be effected by a measure doing more good to the aged than to any other class in the community!"

Neverbend's social order based on the removal of the elderly from society, however, was doomed to failure, if for no other reason than the lack of concordance of chronologic and biologic aging. The first destined to enter the program was Neverbend's close friend, Gabriel Crassweller, a successful and honorable farmer, who, having agreed to the proposal at its conception years earlier, was still a vigorous man in the seventh decade of life. As the day of his confinement approached, the appeal of the concept to him had clearly waned; but, despite increasing depression over the prospect to be faced, he remained prepared to stand by his agreement. Crassweller was not put to test, however; for Britain intervened, removed Neverbend from the island and re-annexed it. Although Neverbend remained committed to the validity of his plan, he became convinced that it was an idea the time for which had not come. In fact, on his journey from Britannula to England aboard the warship, John Bright, he confessed to himself his probable inability to have implemented the law he had so staunchly espoused.

What then should be the role of a prophylactic such as pneumococcal vaccine as it applies to later life in a culture which seeks to maintain its quality? It appears to be safe and effective in adults, and it may be inferred from immunologic studies that protection against infection with the specific pneumococcal types, the antigens of which are in the vaccine, will, for many, be long-lived. The incidence of tetanus in this country has never been very great, probably not exceeding 2 per 100,000 persons per annum before our society was highly urbanized. Retrospective study of pneumococcal bacteremia indicates, conservatively, that the attack rate of this infection exceeds 20 per 100,000 per annum among persons over 60 years of age;[51] and the mortality among those stricken in this age group is greater than 25 percent. If it is reasonable to advocate universal immunization to prevent tetanus, it would seem equally reasonable to immunize those of high risk of death from pneumococcal infection, among them all persons reaching 55 years of age.

A potentially useful addendum to the prophylactic armamentarium of the geriatrician is at hand. Only by its wider use can further knowledge of its potential benefits and limitations be gained. Whether or not such knowledge will be gained rests in large measure in the hands of those whose primary responsibility is the care of the patient.

Acknowledgments. I am deeply indebted to the following collaborators whose diligence, insights and contributions led to the licensure of the contemporary pneumococcal vaccine. Drs. Gerald Schiffman, Mary J. Bonner, Robert M. Douglas, Arnold R.

Saslow, Mr.Boone W. Mora, Drs. William J. Buffaloe, Marvin A. Fried, Ms. Barbara Thompson, Drs. Cyril H. Wyndham, James H. S. Gear, Albert M. Coetzee, Robert D. W. Reid, Hendrik J. Koornhof, Mr. Stanley Hayden-Smith and Mr. Andrew Heyns.

References

1. Heffron, R.: Pneumonia with Special Reference to Pneumococcus Lobar Pneumonia. (Second printing.) Cambridge, MA, Harvard University Press, 1979, (a) pp. 299–307; (b) pp. 557–558.

2. Kovar, M. D.: Health of the elderly and use of health services, Public Hlth. Rep. 92: 9, 1977.

3. Charcot, J. M.: Leçons sur les Maladies des Vieillards et les Maladies Chroniques. Paris, A. Delahaye, 1868.

4. Hourmann and Dechambre: Recherches pour servir à l'histoire des maladies des vieillards, faites a la Salpêtrière. Maladies des organes de la respiration, Arch. gén. Méd. (Paris, 2ᵉSer.) 8: 405, 1835.

5. Hourmann and Dechambre: Respiration chez les vieillards, Ibid., 9: 338, 1835.

6. Hourmann and Dechambre: (3ᵉMémoire). Pneumonie chez les vieillards. Iʳᵉ partie—Caractères anatomiques, Ibid., 10: 269, 1836.

7. Hourmann and Dechambre: (4ᵉMémoire). Pneumonie des vieillards. IIᵉ Partie—Etiologie et symptomatologie, Ibid., 12: 27, 1836.

8. Hourmann and Dechambre: (5ᵉ et dernier Mémoire). Pneumonie des vieillards. (2ᵉPartie.) Symptomatologie. Symptômes généraux, Ibid., 12: 164, 1836.

9. Chatard, J. A.: The leucocytes in acute lobar pneumonia, Johns Hopkins Hosp. Rep. 15: 89, 1910.

10. Zeman, F. D. and Wallach, K.: Pneumonia in the aged. An analysis of one hundred sixty-six cases of its occurrence in patients sixty years old and over, Arch. Int. Med. 77: 678, 1946.

11. Helpern, M. and Rabson, S. M.: Sudden and unexpected natural death—General considerations and statistics, New York State Med. J. 45: 1197, 1945.

12. Denham, M. J. and Goodwin, G. S.: The value of blood cultures in geriatric practice, Age & Ageing 6: 85, 1977.

13. Townsend, C. W. and Coolidge, A., Jr.: The mortality of acute lobar pneumonia. From a study of all the cases of this disease treated at the Massachusetts General Hospital from the first case in 1822 up to the present day, Tr. Am. Climatol. A. 6: 22, 1889.

14. Shattuck, F. C. and Lawrence, C. H.: Acute lobar pneumonia, Boston Med. Surg. J. 178: 245, 1918.

15. Harford, C. G., Leidler, V. and Hara, M.: Effect of the lesion due to influenza virus on the resistance of mice to inhaled pneumococci, J. Exp. Med. 89: 53, 1949.

16. Harford, C. G. and Hara, M.: Pulmonary edema in influenzal pneumonia in the mouse and the relation of fluid in the lung to the inception of pneumococcal pneumonia, J. Exp. Med. 91: 245, 1950.

17. Dhar, S., Shastri, S. R. and Lenora, R. A. K.: Aging and the respiratory system, Med. Clin. North Amer. 60: 1121, 1976.

18. Gardner, A. M. N.: Aspiration of food and vomit, Quart. J. Med. 27: 227, 1958.

19. Phair, J. P., Kauffman, C. A., Bjornson, A. et al.: Host defenses in the aged: evaluation of components of the inflammatory and immune responses, J. Infect. Dis. 138: 67, 1978.

20. Phair, J. P.: Aging and infection: a review, J. Chron. Dis. 32: 535, 1979.

21. Gardner, I. D.: The effect of aging on susceptibility to infection, Rev. Infect. Dis. 2: 801, 1980.

22. Gwaltney, J. M., Jr., Sande, M. A., Austrian, R. et al.: Spread of *Streptococcus pneumoniae* in families. II. Relation of transfer of *S. pneumoniae* to incidence of colds and serum antibody, J. Infect. Dis. 132: 62, 1975.

23. Sutliff, W. D. and Finland, M.: Antipneumococcic immunity reactions in individuals of different ages, J. Exp. Med. 55: 837, 1932.

24. Finland, M. and Sutliff, W. D.: Immunity reactions in human subjects to strains of pneumococci other than types I, II and III, J. Exp. Med. 57: 95, 1933.

25. Austrian, R. and Gold, J.: Pneumococcal bacteremia with special reference to bacteremic pneumococcal pneumonia, Ann. Int. Med. 60: 759, 1964.

26. Mufson, M. A., Kruss, D. M., Wasil, R. E. et al.: Capsular types and outcomes of bacteremic pneumococcal disease in the antibiotic era, Arch. Int. Med. 134: 505, 1974.

27. McGowen, J. E., Barnes, M. W. and Finland, M.: Bacteremia at the Boston City Hospital: ocurrence and mortality during 12 selected years (1935–1972), with special reference to hospital-acquired cases, J. Infect. Dis. 132: 316, 1975.

28. Dowling, H. F. and Lepper, M. H.: The effect of antibiotics (penicillin, aureomycin and terramycin) on the fatality rate and incidence of complications in pneumococcic pneumonia, Am. J. Med. Sci. 222: 396, 1951.

29. Ziskind, M. M., Schwarz, M. I., George, R. B. et al.: Incomplete consolidation in pneumococcal lobar pneumonia complicating pulmonary emphysema, Ann. Int. Med. 72: 835, 1970.

30. Austrian, R.: Of gold and pneumococci. A history of pneumococcal vaccines in South Africa, Tr. Am. Clin. Climat. A. 89: 141, 1977.

31. Schiemann, O. and Casper, W.: Sind die spezifisch präcipitabelen Substanzen der 3 Pneumokokkentypen Haptene?, Ztschr. Hyg. Infektionskr. 108: 220, 1927.

32. Francis, T., Jr. and Tillett, W. S.: Cutaneous reactions in pneumonia. The development of antibodies following the intradermal injection of type-specific polysaccharide, J. Exp. Med. 52: 573, 1930.

33. MacLeod, C. M., Hodges, R. G., Heidelberger, M. et al.: Prevention of pneumococcal pneumonia by immunization with specific capsular polysaccharides, J. Exp. Med. 82: 445, 1945.

34. Heidelberger, M., di Lapi, M. M., Siegel, M. et al.: Persistence of antibodies in human subjects injected with pneumococcal polysaccharides, J. Immunol. 65: 535, 1950.

35. Austrian, R., Douglas, R. M., Schiffman, G. et al.: Prevention of pneumococcal pneumonia by vaccination, Tr. Assoc. Am. Physicians 89: 184, 1976.

36. Smit, P., Oberholzer, D., Hayden-Smith, S. et al.: Protective efficacy of pneumococcal polysaccharide vaccines, J.A.M.A. 238: 2613, 1977.

37. Francis, T., Jr., Korns, R. F., Voight, B. S. et al.: An evaluation of the 1954

poliomyelitis vaccine trials. Summary Report, Am. J. Public Health 45: Suppl., 1955.

38. Kaufman, P.: Pneumonia in old age. Active immunization against pneumonia with pneumococcus polysaccharide; results of a six year study, Arch. Int. Med. 79: 518, 1947.

39. Thomsen, O. and Kettel, K.: Die Stärke der menschlichen Isogglutinine und entsprechender Blutkörperchenrezeptoren in verschieden Lebensaltern, Ztschr. Immunitätsforsch Exp. Therapie 63: 72, 1929.

40. Center for Disease Control: MMWR Annual Summary 1979. Vol. 28, No. 54, Sept. 1980. U.S. Dept of Health and Human Services Publication No. (CDC) 80-8241. Washington, D.C., U.S. Govt. Printing Office.

41. Ruben, F. L., Nagel, J. and Fireman, P.: Antibody responses in the elderly to tetanus-diphtheria (TD) immunization, Am. J. Epidemiol. 108: 145, 1978.

42. Ammann, A. J., Schiffman, G. and Austrian, R.: The antibody responses to pneumococcal cpsular polysaccharides in aged individuals, Proc. Soc. Exp. Biol. Med. 164: 312, 1980.

43. Radl, J., Sepers, J. M., Skvaril, F. et al: Immunoglobulin patterns in humans over 95 years of age, Clin. Exp. Immunol. 22: 84, 1975.

44. Borgoño, J. M., McLean, A. A., Vella, P. P. et al.: Vaccination and revaccination with polyvalent pneumococcal polysaccharide vaccines in adults and infants, Proc. Soc. Exp. Biol. Med. 157: 48, 1978.

45. Broome, C. V., Facklam, R. R. and Fraser, D. W.: Pneumococcal disease after pneumococcal vaccination. An alternative method to estimate the efficacy of pneumococcal vaccine, N. Engl. J. Med. 303: 549, 1980.

46. Osler, W.: The Principles and Practice of Medicine. (First Ed.) New York, D. Appleton and Co., 1892, p. 511.

47. Osler, W.: The Principles and Practice of Medicine. (Third Ed.) New York, D. Appleton and Co., 1898, pp. 108–109.

48. Osler, W.: The Fixed Period, in Aequanimitas with other addresses to Medical Students, Nurses and Practitioners of Medicine. (Third Ed.) Philadelphia, P. Blakiston Son & Co., Inc., 1932, p. 373.

49. Cushing, H.: The Life of Sir William Osler. Oxford, Clarendon Press, 1925, Vol. 1, pp. 664–674.

50. Trollope, A.: The Fixed Period. Leipzig, B. Tauchnitz, 1882.

51. Filice, G. A., Darby, C P. and Fraser, D. W.: Pneumococcal bacteremia in Charleston County, South Carolina, Am. J. Epidemiol. 112: 828, 1980.

11

Microbiology and Clinical Medicine—A Personal View

Ninetieth anniversaries are seldom events to be celebrated with more than passing interest. Had the year been 1981, I should doubtless have taken this opportunity, bestowed upon me by the Infectious Diseases Society of America, to signalize the discovery of the pneumococcus by Pasteur and by Sternberg, for this organism has played a noteworthy role in the history of infectious diseases and of biology. It has not been overlooked, however, in this week's programs; and rather than preempt the centennial of its initial isolation, I shall avail myself of the privilege of addressing this audience by considering some contemporary aspects of the care of the infected patient. The last thirty years, like those of the late nineteenth century, have been characterized by profound changes both in microbiology and in the clinical management of infectious diseases. It seems fitting that this occasion may serve as a time to review some of these changes and to take stock of the problems that still confront us. The views to be expressed are personal ones, and there will doubtless be some among you who will take exception to them. This likelihood notwithstanding, they will have served their purpose if they are provocative of thought and action which will lead to improvement in the care of the infected patient, whatever the path of evolution from our present condition.

Infections still constitute the major portion of illnesses today. The family study of Dingle and his associates[1] indicates that 72% of the morbidity among the individuals observed could be classified as due to infections. Most of the illness seen was mild and self-limited, although occasional ones of greater severity were noted. How well are infections handled in medical practice today? Specific answers to this question are difficult to obtain. We are all aware of the potent antibacterial agents now available and of their not infrequent administration to patients on the basis of inappropriate indications. Although they are devoid neither of toxic nor of sensitizing properties, many predominantly affect metabolic reactions of the parasite with relatively little physiologic impact on the host. This fact may account for the relative impunity with which

they may be administered for short periods to many patients without serious
untoward reaction. Such a state of affairs, however, promotes indiscriminate
use and leads patients to seek antibiotic therapy whether or not it is appropriate. It is an interesting paradox that, having obtained a group of potent and
effective drugs, physicians fail frequently today to use discriminatingly the
available laboratory facilities and that certain helpful laboratory procedures
have been largely abandoned.

The optimal use of antimicrobial drugs requires the establishment of a precise etiologic diagnosis whenever circumstances permit. Although many
clinical illnesses present features that are sufficiently typical to enable the physician to make a correct diagnosis, even the most astute physician may err;
and to fail to make use of laboratory facilities when they are available is to
provide less than optimal care. Careful studies of such a common illness as
pharyngitis have shown that the chance of diagnosing clinically the presence
or absence of a streptococcal infection is no better than 70%.[2] To give all patients with sore throats penicillin will certainly lead to the unnecessary sen-
sitization of some; such an occurrence is not too infrequent. Although access
to laboratory facilities may be limited in office practice, they are readily available in most, if not all hospitals. How well attuned are physicians to their use?
Our recent attempts to establish the bacterial etiology of pneumonia suggest
that our present educational efforts are falling short of the desideratum. In a
retrospective study of 500 hospitalized cases of clinically diagnosed pneumonia at an institution with a staff of interns and residents, only 70% of the
patients had cultures of sputum and blood and of these, 25% were from specimens obtained after the administration of antimicrobial drugs. In another hospital, at which 210 deaths attributed to pneumonia were analyzed, 56%
of those who died had had cultures of sputum and 30% had had cultures of
blood; of the sputum cultures, only a quarter were obtained before antibacterial therapy. Although it is recognized that the identification of some potential pathogens in expectorated respiratory secretions does not establish
their causal role in the disease of the lungs, careful microscopic examination,
with attention to cytology as well as to bacteria, and culture of sputum can
often provide information essential to the welfare of the patient. The observation of Gill[3] on the rising mortality from Friedländer's pneumonia after the
replacement of sulfonamides by penicillin is in accord with this view. These
limited but precise observations, together with other personal experiences and
conversations with colleagues, are indicative that efforts to educate physicians
in the management of infectious diseases have not been wholly successful.

The teaching of microbiology and of infectious disease has undergone significant alterations in the past three decades. With the studies of Marjory
Stephenson[4] in the 1920's and later with those of Fildes, Knight, Woods, and

others, microbiology began to change from a predominantly descriptive science to one dealing with many of the fundamental aspects of all biology. The growing recognition of the many similarities of all forms of life and the ease of adaptability of bacteria and viruses to studies of many basic biologic problems have made possible striking advances in genetics, biochemistry, pharmacology, and immunology. Medicine may take just pride in its contributions to biologic knowledge. Much of the information gleaned from such studies is highly relevant to medical practice and has rightly become a part of the medical curriculum. Its volume, however, has created a problem in the organization of curricula without extending their already imposing length, and much of what was taught in courses of microbiology about the isolation and identification of pathogenic microorganisms must now be encompassed in a shorter span of time. As a result, the student frequently comes to his introductory clinical period with less experience in diagnostic microbiology than he did several decades ago. At a conference held in 1963 on the teaching of infectious diseases at the Center for Communicable Diseases sponsored by the United States Public Health Service,[5] there was general acceptance that this change was inevitable and that transmission of the newer fundamental knowledge to the medical student was essential to his education as a modern physician. However, it was also stressed that, whenever possible, teaching and laboratory experience in microbiology should be designed to stress its relevance to the clinical practice. To this end, it is desirable that some member of a department of microbiology hold a doctorate in medicine so that he can bring to the students the perspective of the physician. In his absence, it is helpful to enlist such an individual from another department to aid in teaching. The course should also acquaint the student with those organisms which make up the microflora of the human body, with the more common pathogenic bacteria, and with the basic techniques essential for their isolation. Emphasis on the precise identification of most microbes and on many of the details of microbial classification will have to be diminished because of the limitations of time.

To compensate for these alterations in courses of basic microbiology, other mechanisms must be devised to teach undergraduate and postdoctoral students both the clinical and the laboratory aspects essential to the intelligent management of infectious disorders. To do so requires careful scrutiny of a number of trends in recent years that have rendered the task more complex. Restructure of the medical curriculum to make it resemble more closely that of other forms of graduate education, administrative transfer of clinical microbiological laboratories from the departments of medicine and pediatrics to those of clinical pathology, and the closing of isolation facilities have all had their impact.

Modification of the medical curriculum has been a major preoccupation of medical faculties in recent years. This has been so because changes in high school and college education have provided students with a better background in biology; for them we need to eliminate material duplicated in preclinical courses. The length of medical education and its increasing cost have provided another stimulus to seek ways of shortening it. In addition, greater freedom of choice in the selection of course material has been urged by students. The impetus of these factors has led to the development of "core" curricula in a number of schools with marked curtailment of required classes and much additional time for electives. Efforts to permit early specialization in medicine by the development of educational "tracks" have also received considerable attention. The goals are admirable in seeking to provide more physicians at lower cost to society, physicians who, through some investigative effort of their own, are better able to think and to practice more critically. Faculties have the responsibility, however, of assuring that all who are awarded a doctorate in medicine have sufficient breadth of knowledge to recognize the nature of the clinical problems they will encounter subsequently, even if only to know when to enlist the aid of others in the care of patients for which they lack the necessary expertise. There are hazards, as Romano has pointed out,[6] in "requiring early commitment and thus reducing options early in the intellectual and professional life of the student, making more difficult the possibility of intelligent choice from the wide range of opportunities throughout the undergraduate period. Medicine is a rich and varied menu." Like many subspecialties of medicine, the study of infectious disease crosses all clinical departmental lines, and every student should have adequate grounding in this subject, whatever his ultimate aim. The fact that many infections today are treatable disorders when they are properly managed gives added importance to this need.

With the changes in the curriculum in microbiology, a greater responsibility for the teaching of both laboratory and clinical aspects of infectious disease has become the lot of departments of medicine and pediatrics. Introductory courses, required or elective, with interdepartmental participation of the faculties of medicine, pediatrics, microbiology, and pathology can be a useful means of preparing the student for further clinical experience. The value of the course can be augmented by the inclusion of laboratory exercises which emphasize, in addition to fundamental aspects of host-parasite relationships, those diagnostic procedures which the physician can do himself to facilitate and to expedite diagnosis. The inclusion of a limited number of unknowns for identification in the laboratory, while viewed by some students as a threat, provides experience in educationally fashionable "problem solving" and, concomitantly, the opportunity to learn some facts without which problem solving becomes a sterile exercise. At the risk of beating a tired horse, it is urged that the proper technique of performing the Gram stain be taught so that improperly made preparations will be recognized and attempts to draw conclusions from them will be avoided. Too often precipitated gentian violet is still interpreted by the inexperienced or unwary as indicating the presence of gram-positive bacteria. For the infected patient, the proper interpretation of the Gram-stained body fluid or secretion is as important as the correct reading of the electrocardiogram of the patient with heart disease.

The advent of antimicrobial drugs and of an increasing number of effective vaccines has brought about significant alterations in the management of the infected patient. Hospitals for communicable disease have virtually ceased to exist in this country, and most general hospitals have closed their isolation units. These changes have had their impact on both patient care and teaching. Initial overoptimism concerning the ability of antimicrobial drugs to control infection and the lack of a centralized area in which good isolation technique can be practiced and taught have been contributory factors to the present day problem of nosocomial infection, the magnitude of which is well known to this audience. I suggest that there is a definite place today for one or more small isolation units in many general hospitals, especially in those engaged in teaching. Such a unit can set proper standards of environmental hygiene, which can then be translated to other areas of the hospital where patients with potentially communicable disease are housed. This latter aim is furthered if house staff, students, and nurses rotate through the unit. The value of an isolation unit will be enhanced if a small bacteriologic laboratory is made a part of it. It need be neither large nor elaborate, and might consist only of a small incubator, a refrigerator for media, appropriate stains, a microscope, a table centrifuge, and the usual utilities of a laboratory. Here, with adequate supervision, students and resident staff can acquire some much needed first-hand experience with the capabilities of diagnostic microbiology. Although it may be objected that economic considerations will preclude such activities, there is a strong likelihood that more intelligent use of the diagnostic microbiological laboratory by those who have had such experience will offset the costs incurred. It is to be hoped that the recently recorded experience of one general hospital at which more urine cultures than urinalyses were performed[7] could be modified.

If centralized bedside teaching of infectious disease is not possible, it must be carried out on each hospital unit where infected patients are located, aided, when appropriate, by consultation with those who have a special interest in this area of medicine. Although maintenance of adequate standards of isolation is often more difficult when this situation prevails, their use, when indicated, should receive adequate emphasis. This need is especially great in intensive care units, both medical and surgical, where many vulnerable patients, some infected, may be in close proximity to one another. Facilities adequate to permit simple laboratory procedures, including the staining and examination of slides, should be easily available to those immediately concerned with the patients.

In the teaching of infectious disease, as in all areas of clinical medicine, there is a critical need today to stress the methods of history-taking and physical diagnosis to balance the increasing reliance on technical procedures performed by persons other than the attending physician. It is a curious paradox that incoming students, restive during the preclinical years, with their emphasis on the laboratory and their denial of contact with patients, tend to lean so heavily on the laboratory once at the bedside. Time spent in the careful taking of a history provides an opportunity for physician and patient to know one another better and the record should include not only the conventional "Present Illness" and "Review of Systems," but also a reasonably detailed social history providing insights into the patient's past and present occupations, social adjustment, and habits. Confidence is inspired by compassionate interest on the part of the physician, and clues to diagnosis are often forthcoming. History-taking and physical diagnosis are the basic tools of the physician and are acquired only with meticulous attention to detail and with repetition. It cannot be denied that much of the work required to develop the necessary skills is boring to students and teachers alike, but they can be learned in no other way, and the ultimate rewards are great. It is easier to obtain an X-ray of the chest than to carry out and record the inspection, palpation, percussion, and auscultation thereof, but I have seen at least four instances in which an erroneous clinical diagnosis of pneumonia was concurred in by the radiologist when both the history and physical examination pointed clearly to the true nature of the illness, tuberculous pleurisy with effusion. How often today does one find mention of the position of the trachea and a description of thoracic and of diaphragmatic motion in routine physical examinations? A brief review of charts on several teaching services suggests that there is room for significant improvement. As concerned physicians, we must teach and practice that laboratories, no matter how helpful, can err at times; thus each physician must develop sufficient confidence in his own abilities to evaluate an illness and to question unusual or discordant laboratory findings when they occur. It is not uncommon for physicians to ask the clinical microbiologic laboratory to make value judgments regarding the significance of results when, in fact, it is the responsibility of those who care directly for the patient.

It is important that physicians learn that the collection of specimens for microbiologic examinations is a personal responsibility; and that, when delegated to others, it must be to individuals known to be adequately trained to carry out the proper procedures. Sputum to be cultured should be produced by the patient in the presence of one able to assure that the secretions are indeed expectorated. All too often contents of a container left at the bedside to be sent later to the laboratory will be saliva. Proper instruction in cleansing technique must be given to those charged with the collection of urine for culture. And the value of taking media to the bedside for a variety of cultural procedures should be stressed. Labeling of the specimen should provide the laboratory with as precise and accurate a clinical diagnosis as can be reached through the history and physical examination so that the proper procedures may be employed. The frequent absence or imprecision of such information is the bane of the laboratory and has led one British microbiologist to write a paper plaintively entitled "Why Teach Microbiology?"[8] Requests for viral studies are often of a nature that precludes genuine laboratory assistance because of their lack of precision. The physician seeking help of this kind must know what viral agents are potential causes of a given infection and must indicate them when asking for assistance. The need to assay the level of antibody in two or more serum specimens to arrive at a serologic diagnosis of a viral or other infection is all too frequently overlooked. Single requests for "febrile agglutinins," an unhappy term to those with a concern for the usage of English, rarely lead to rewarding results in the diagnosis of salmonellosis or of other infections and more often promote confusion. Better instruction in the principles of serodiagnosis is clearly required.

Constant emphasis in undergraduate and postdoctoral education should be given to restraint in the immediate adminstration of antimicrobial drugs to febrile patients, many of whom have self-limited illnesses not amenable to medications currently extant. Some patients, as I have learned from painful personal experience, may recover in spite of the ministrations of the physician rather than because of them. As is true of all maladies, the physician must make a value judgment of a febrile disease and an assessment as to whether or not the fever is of infectious origin. Those of us who received our introduction to medicine before antimicrobial drugs were available in profusion had the experience of seeing many patients survive febrile illness and became aware that fever per se did not necessarily imply a fatal prognosis. We lived with patients, often in poor general health, in whom malaria was produced as therapy for syphilis of the central nervous system and who were considered to have had adequate treatment only after they had 50 hours of fever of 104°F or more. Such experiences have a tempering effect on one's outlook on fever. To state the foregoing is not to imply that one should treat lightly significant elevations of temperature, but only that such a finding, considered by itself, should not be an immediate indication for overly hasty and indiscriminate therapy. There is need also for a reorientation of thinking with regard to the implications of high fever and hypotension. By many, these signs are now equated with the diagnosis of "gram-negative septicemia," an unfortunate term which tends to eliminate consideration of other diagnostic possibilities that give rise to similar clinical findings, and which leads at times to inappropriate or overly heroic treatment.

Teaching of the use of antimicrobial drugs should stress pharmacologic principles and the choice of the least toxic and least allergenic regimen adequate to deal with the problem at hand. All antibacterial drugs alter to some degree the microbial flora of the host, and the changes are not always effected with impunity. There is well-documented evidence that the use of large doses of penicillin in the treatment of pneumonia is more likely to be followed by superinfection than when adequate but smaller amounts are employed.[9] In light of these findings, the tendency of some to increase the dose in direct relation to the height of the patient's temperature seems unwarranted. I have been struck also in recent years by the extraordinary increase in the use of ampicillin when treatment with penicillin G, a penicillinase-resistant penicillin, or an unrelated antibiotic was indicated. I suspect that ampicillin, which I have facetiously termed today's "decerebrate antibiotic," will soon be replaced by cephalexin which, unlike ampicillin, has the additional attribute of being resistant to beta lactamases. If combinations of antibiotics are to be used, one should always be able to defend the rationale for the ones selected, and the potential antagonism by bacteriostatic agents of those drugs which act by inhibiting synthesis of the bacterial cell wall should be familiar to all. The observation that a bacterium is sensitive in vitro to two or more drugs is not in itself the final determinant that these drugs should be administered concomitantly, and the decision to resort to polypharmacy must be soundly based.

The microbiologic laboratory plays a pivotal role in the care of the infected patient. When it is a division of clinical pathology, every effort must be made to assure close and continuous communication between the clinical and laboratory staffs. This goal may be rendered difficult in large hospitals in which the laboratory is geographically remote from the areas in which patients are housed and may require special efforts on the part of those concerned. It is useful to have joint appointments of one or more clinicians to the laboratory staff and to provide opportunities to house officers and medical students to spend some time, required or elective, in the laboratory. Interplay of this kind also provides the opportunity for the staff of the laboratory to call attention to the misuse of its facilities and to lessen the demand for potentially unrewarding tests. There is mutual advantage to be gained from assuring the proper collection of specimens, their accurate labeling and prompt delivery to the laboratory, and the expeditious reporting of results.

The introduction of quality control into laboratories of clinical microbiology is of relatively recent origin and marks an important and welcome advance. The efforts of the College of American Pathologists[10, 11] in fostering this activity are to be applauded, and all such laboratories should be encouraged to participate in its program. In this fashion, shortcomings can be identified and corrected, and awareness of the newer methods of diagnostic microbiology can be heightened. Among these are developments in the isolation of anaerobic bacteria, the more precise identification of the Enterobacteriaceae and the standardization of antimicrobial sensitivity tests. Caution should be exercised, however, in discarding time-tested techniques in favor of newer but less precise methods. There is little question but that the ability to identify the pneumococcus has declined significantly with the abandonment of serotyping of this organism and that this step has been a significant contributory factor to present misconceptions about the incidence of pneumococcal disease. It is of interest that typing sera for all pneumococcal types, including a concentrated polyvalent globulin that contains antibody to all 82 pneumococcal types, can be obtained only from Denmark. This latter reagent will permit immediate identification of pneumococci in sputum and body fluids and is invaluable in the rapid diagnosis of pneumococcal meningitis. The capsular precipitin or quellung reaction can be applied also to the identification of *Haemophilus influenzae*, some types of meningococci, and strains of *Klebsiella pneumoniae*. Its potential value in the recognition of outbreaks of nosocomial infection caused by *Klebsiella* remains largely unexploited.

The clinical microbiologic laboratory can serve not only to provide information necessary for the care of patients but also as a focal point for essential epidemiologic activities within the hospital community. It should monitor the sterility of surgical equipment and those devices now used so widely in the treatment of respiratory disease. In addition, the increasing availability of computerized analyses of laboratory results should facilitate the work of the hospital committee on infections and of the nurse epidemiologist. Data concerning the sensitivity of specific organisms to antimicrobial drugs collated in similar fashion can provide useful information to the clinical staff in formulating the therapy that is potentially most beneficial before specific information is available in a given infection. Last but not least, the laboratory staff should encourage contact with clinicians and provide opportunities for the instruction of all who seek it. Willingness to support decentralized facilities as an aid to teaching is an integral part of this effort in educational institutions.

In the final analysis, the success of medical education and of the medical care of infections is dependent upon the attitude that places the welfare of the patient above all else. The quality of care, teaching, and research all suffer when this aim is not the primary one of all concerned with the health of others. To achieve this goal requires sufficient breadth and depth of knowledge, the discipline of high standards, meticulous attention to detail, and the fostering of an awareness that much of medicine is a "do-it-yourself" operation. In an era of rapid changes in knowledge, technology, and education, success will be achieved as we modify our approaches if these time-tested verities are borne in mind.

References

1. Dingle, J. H., Badger, G. F., Feller, A. E., Hodges, R. G., Jordan, W. S., Jr., Rammelkamp, C. H., Jr. A study of illness in a group of Cleveland families. I. Plan of study and certain general observations. Amer. J. Hy. 58: 16–30, 1953.

2. Breese, B. B., Disney, F. A. The accuracy of diagnosis of beta streptococcal infections. J. Pediat. 44: 670–673, 1954.

3. Gill, R. J. Treatment of Friedländer's pneumonia. Amer. J. Med. Sci. 221: 5–9, 1950.

4. Stephenson, M. Bacterial metabolism. Longmans, Green and Co., London, 1930.

5. Tager, M., Sellers, T. F., Jr., Mastin, D. S. [ed.] Proceedings of the national conference on the teaching of infectious disease in U.S. medical schools, Atlanta, Georgia, March 11–13, 1963. J. Med. Educ. 39: 1–116, 1964.

6. Romano, J. The elimination of the internship—an act of retrogression. Amer. J. Psychiat. 126: 1565–1576, 1970.

7. Griner, P. F., Liptzin, B. Use of the laboratory in a teaching hospital. Implications for patient care, education, and hospital costs. Ann. Int. Med. 75: 157–163, 1971.

8. Boycott, J. A. Why teach microbiology? Lancet 1: 724–725, 1969.

9. Louria, D. B., Brayton, R. G. The efficacy of penicillin regimens with observations on the frequency of superinfection. J.A.M.A. 186: 987–990, 1963.

10. Gavan, T. L., King, J. W. An evaluation of the microbiology portions of the 1969 basic, comprehensive, and special College of American Pathologists proficiency testing surveys. Amer. J. Clin. Path. 54: 514–520, 1970.

11. Barnett, R. N. Conference on the medical usefulness of microbiology, Amer. J. Clin. Path. 54: 521–530, 1970.

12

The Syndrome of Pneumococcal Endocarditis, Meningitis, and Rupture of the Aortic Valve

The advent of an effective prophylactic and therapeutic agent may alter significantly both the incidence and etiology of a given anatomical lesion and such may be the effect of penicillin upon aortic valvular disease. As a result of its use in the treatment of early syphilis, luetic disease of the aortic valve is seen with lessening frequency, and it is altogether possible that the widespread employment of penicillin as a prophylactic against rheumatic fever may result in a decrease in aortic valvular disease of rheumatic origin. Concomitant with the decline of two of the major causes of aortic valvular disease, lesions of other etiologies will acquire relatively greater significance and paradoxically, antibiotics and notably penicillin can be responsible for the emergence of one of these. By preventing the premature death of patients with pneumococcal endocarditis, a hitherto almost uniformly fatal disorder, penicillin enables some of these individuals to recover from their bacterial infection even though they may suffer in a number of instances rupture of the aortic valve as a result of bacterial damage prior to therapy. Such a sequence of events has been observed in the past decade in eight patients, and they comprise the subject of the present report. Before they are described, however, a brief review of knowledge relating to the clinical picture they present may be pertinent.

Recognition of the association of pneumonia, endocarditis and meningitis is not new. Perhaps the first to relate these three lesions to one another was the Austrian pathologist, Heschl, who described, in 1862, autopsies upon five patients who had died with this triad of abnormalities.[1] In 1881, the year pneumococcus was discovered, Osler wrote in a paper entitled "Infectious (So-Called Ulcerative) Endocarditis": "Meningitis is a very rare complication of pneumonia and may occur apart from endocarditis; but in a case of inflammation of the lungs, particularly if the apex is involved (in three out of four such instances I found the upper part of the lung affected), the development of an irregular temperature with cerebral symptoms should suggest the possibility of endocardial mischief, with secondary meningeal inflammation."[2]

To the French physician, Netter, however, must go much of the credit for elucidating the pathogenesis of pneumococcal endocarditis. In 1886, he reviewed eighty-two cases of endocarditis associated with pneumonia including two observed by himself.[3] He demonstrated the similarity of the organism isolated from endocardial vegetations to that recovered from the lung in seven fatal cases and grew pneumococcus from the blood of a patient shown subsequently to have endocarditis of the tricuspid valve. By traumatizing the aortic valve of the rabbit with a stylet passed down the carotid artery, he was able to produce experimental endocarditis in this animal following subsequent infection with pneumococcus. He pointed out the predilection of pneumococcus for localization upon the aortic valve whether normal or previously diseased and the relative frequency with which it attacks the valves of the right side of the heart. He was impressed also with the high incidence of meningitis in those with this cardiac disorder.

In 1904, Preble reviewed again the subject of pneumococcal endocarditis, adding fifty cases to those studied earlier by Netter and emphasizing the clinical aspects of the disease.[4] He noted its more frequent occurrence in older individuals, its variable duration with death occurring on the average a month following onset, and its complication by meningitis in approximately three-fifths of the cases. One additional observation, made also by Netter, is noteworthy. In twenty of the patients, an afebrile interval was observed following the period of pneumonia and prior to the recrudescence of fever associated with endocarditis. In a temperature chart shown in Netter's paper,[3] defervescence occurred at the usual time of crisis in pneumococcal pneumonia only to be followed in three to four days by a return of fever. The phenomenon points to the probable inefficacy of antibody as an aid to the eradication of infection of the endocardium which view is supported by later evidence. Thomas and O'Hara described fatality following the administration of large amounts of specific antiserum to a patient with type I pneumococcal endocarditis.[5] In this patient, fever and bacteremia recurred following the artificial induction of crisis with passive immunization and persisted despite repeated injections of antibody. Of interest also are the observations of Wadsworth and Sickles upon endocarditis in horses immunized with live pneumococcal vaccines.[6] Not only did these animals develop endocarditis at a time when circulating type-specific antibody was demonstrable, but in the course of continuing infection, the selective effect of capsular antibody upon the bacterial population of the infected animal led to the appearance, at times, of noncapsulated pneumococci in the circulation. Because natural recovery from pneumococcal infection is dependent almost wholly upon phagocytosis of the invading organisms by polymorphonuclear leukocytes, these observations point to a local failure of the phagocytic mechanism in endocardial infection. If this inference is a correct one, then recovery following treatment with other than a bactericidal agent will not be likely. The failure of the bacteriostatic sulfonamides to modify the uniformly fatal outcome in pneumococcal endocarditis is consistent with this view, and Heffron's statement in his monograph of 1939[7] that it is doubtful that an authenticated instance of recovery from the disease had ever been reported remained largely true until penicillin became available for the treatment of it.

From the foregoing discussion, it is evident that the association of pneumococcal endocarditis and meningitis has long been recognized and that until recently death from infection has been the outcome for those so afflicted. The introduction of a drug bactericidal for pneumococcus has modified significantly the clinical course of the syndrome; and, by making possible survival from infection, penicillin has allowed the recognition of a new group of patients with aortic insufficiency.

This most recent chapter in this history of pneumococcal endocarditis begins on February 1, 1946, when Case #1, a 46 year old black male was admitted because of his irrational mental state to Sydenham Hospital in Baltimore. Four weeks previously he had developed pneumonia for the treatment of which his physician had prescribed a sulfonamide. He had improved gradually until the day before hospitalization when his temperature rose and he complained of a stiff neck. Twenty-fours hours later he became delirious and was brought to the hospital.

Physical examination at the time of admission showed an acutely ill, delirious man with a temperature of 104.8°F. The classical signs of meningeal irritation were present. Evidence of pneumonia was not detected. The heart was of normal size and the cardiac sounds were clear. Aside from a soft systolic murmur audible just to the left of the sternum, no auscultatory abnormalities were recorded. The pulse rate was 120 and the blood pressure 148/90.

Examination of the spinal fluid confirmed promptly the clinical impression of meningitis, and pneumococcus Type XIV was grown both from the blood and from the spinal fluid. The serologic test for syphilis was positive in the blood but negative in the spinal fluid.

Treatment with sulfadiazine intravenously and with penicillin intravenously and intrathecally was instituted promptly and over a period of ten days the patient's mental state improved gradually. His temperature returned to normal

on the eighteenth hospital day, but his course was marked later by several episodes of fever and of pulmonary infiltration which, in retrospect, may have
resulted from pulmonary infarction.

On March 28, the heart was noted for the first time to be enlarged and an
aortic diastolic murmur was heard along the left sternal border. Because the
patient's serologic test for syphilis was persistently positive, he was thought to
have syphilitic aortic insufficiency which had been overlooked at the time of
admission; and he was transferred to the Johns Hopkins Hospital for further
study. There the diagnosis of aortic insufficiency of luetic origin was also
deemed likely and the patient was discharged without evidence of cardiac failure on May 8.

He returned to the Johns Hopkins Hospital eighteen days later complaining
of swollen ankles and of nocturnal shortness of breath of a week's duration.
Signs of cardiac failure were present. Digitalization by the oral route was begun but the patient died suddenly and unexpectedly the night of admission to
the hospital. The final clinical impression was syphilitic aortic insufficiency.

Autopsy performed four hours after death yielded findings surprising to
those who had cared for the patient though in retrospect they should not have
been. The aorta was normal. The heart was enlarged but showed none of the
stigmata of treponemal infection. Instead, a perforation of the left cusp of
the aortic valve (Figure 1) 6 mm. in diameter was present which, on microscopic examination, showed at its margins remnants of a healing vegetation.
The pathological diagnosis was healed bacterial endocarditis with perforation
of an aortic cusp.

Only one day after the death of the patient whose history has been recounted, Case #2, a 65 year old black male, was admitted to the medical
wards of the Johns Hopkins Hospital with meningitis and bacteremia caused
by pneumococcus Type XII and signs of aortic insufficiency. With yesterday's
lesson still fresh in their minds, the clinical diagnosis of pneumococcal endocarditis was made by the medical staff; and when the patient died two and a
half months after his initial hospitalization, the clinical impression was confirmed at autopsy.

Since the time of the deaths of the two patients just described, six additional cases of pneumococcal endocarditis with rupture of the aortic valve
have been recognized (Table 1). Among the total of eight patients, all but one
were males and all were over the age of forty. Seven were hospitalized with
clinical and laboratory evidence of meningitis and the eighth patient had a
well-documented history of meningitis two months prior to the pneumococcal
infection during the course of which aortic insufficiency was recognized for
the first time. Six of the eight patients had no evidence of cardiac disease
when examined initially; but two, one of whom had late syphilis, had signs of

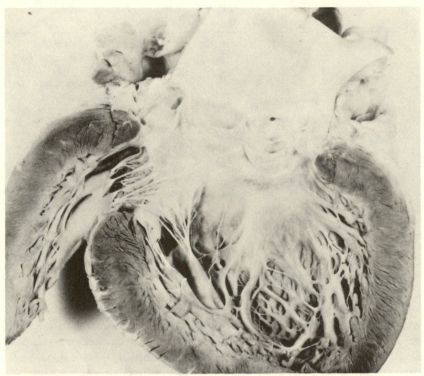

Fig. 1.—Photograph of the heart in Case #1 showing the perforation of a cusp of the aortic valve.

aortic insufficiency when first seen. In those lacking the murmur of aortic insufficiency when hospitalized, it was detected first on the third to fifty-fifth day following admission. It is not improbable, however, that its presence in some patients might have been noted earlier had it been sought more carefully.

All eight patients were treated with penicillin when hospitalized with meningitis though in varying amounts and by different routes of administration. The dosage ranged from 240,000 units to 60,000,000 units per day. Intrathecal therapy was employed in the treatment of three patients and sulfonamides were administered concomitant with penicillin to four. Case #8 had an unusual course. He was hospitalized elsewhere with purulent meningitis in October, 1954, and recovered following treatment with penicillin though the causative organism was not isolated. No evidence of cardiac disease was noted at this time. Two months later, he was admitted to the medical wards with lobar pneumonia and bacteremia caused by pneumococcus Type III at

Table 1. *Clinical and Laboratory Data Pertaining to Eight Patients with Pneumococcal Endocarditis and Rupture of the Aortic Valve*

Case #	Age	Sex	Race	Blood Culture	CSF Culture	STS	Detection of Aortic Insufficiency Days after Adm.	Duration of Life. Days after Detection of Aortic Insufficiency
1	47	M	B	Pnc 14	Pnc 14	+	55	60
2	65	M	B	Pnc 12	Pnc 12	−	On admn.	75
3	50	M	B	Pnc 22	Pnc 22	+	On admn.	41
4	43	F	B	Pnc 12	Pos. Smear	±	3	8
5	74	M	W	Pnc 14	Pnc 14	?	20	1
6	44	M	W	Pnc 8	Pnc 8	−	19	185
7	55	M	W	Pnc 18	Pnc 18	−	3	135+
8	40	M	B	Pnc 3	−	−	12	565+

which time his heart was again described as normal. He was treated with tetracycline for nine days, the last two of which he was afebrile. Three days following cessation of antibacterial therapy, an aortic diastolic murmur was heard though the patient's temperature remained normal. He was given additional treatment with penicillin and remained free of signs of infection.

Development of altered circulatory dynamics after rupture of the aortic valve has been followed with recorded observations in one patient, Case #7. The patient, a 55 year old white male, was admitted to the hospital with pneumonia involving the right middle lobe and with meningitis caused by pneumococcus Type XVIII. Three days after admission, a faint murmur of aortic insufficiency was heard for the first time. Five days later, recordings were made of the patient's ballistocardiogram, carotid pulse curve and stethophonogram. The only abnormality detected was the presence of the aortic diastolic murmur (Figure 2). One month later, little change from the initial tracings was evident, but four months after hospitalization, alterations in the ballistocardiogram, carotid pulse curve and stethophonogram, all characteristic of aortic insufficiency, were noted. When last examined, the patient was in severe cardiac failure aggravated by multiple episodes of pulmonary infarction.

Death in the six fatal cases occurred from one day to six months after the signs of aortic insufficiency were first recognized and from eleven days to seven months following initial hospitalization for pneumococcal infection. In all instances, the fatal outcome was preceded by myocardial failure. Two pa-

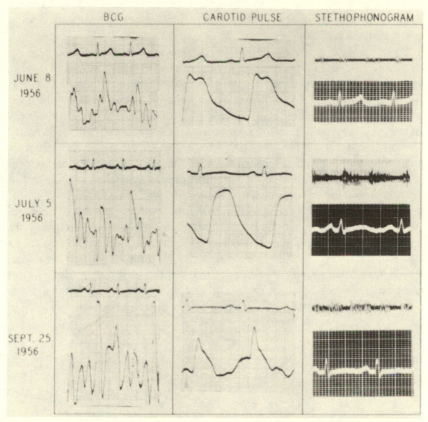

Fig. 2.—Serial ballistocardiograms, carotid pulse tracings, and stethophonograms recorded at Erb's point of Case #7. The tracings show the increasing intensity and duration of the aortic diastolic murmur, a progressive increase in the amplitude of the systolic complexes of the ballistocardiogram and, in the latest record, a shortening of the time from onset to attainment of the peak systolic pressure in the carotid pulse wave, all characteristic findings of progressive aortic insufficiency. All EKG tracings for timing the cardiac cycle are lead 2.

tients, Case #7 and Case #8, were known to be alive four months and twenty months respectively after the development of aortic insufficiency though the former was in severe cardiac failure.

Four of the patients who succumbed were examined post mortem and all showed evidence of healed bacterial endocarditis of the aortic valve with rupture or perforation of a leaflet. Of the four, two had had positive serologic tests for syphilis and two an aortic diastolic murmur at the time of hospitalization. The only patient with both these findings presented pathologic changes compatible with those of healed bacterial endocarditis superimposed upon a preexisting luetic lesion.

From the data reviewed, it appears that the syndrome of pneumococcal endocarditis, meningitis and rupture of the aortic valve, while uncommon, is not rare; for it has been observed in approximately twenty per cent of the patients with pneumococcal meningitis seen by the writer in the past decade. The presence of pneumococcal endocarditis may be anticipated in a quarter to a third of patients hospitalized with pneumococcal meningitis and will be detected perhaps more often if this association is borne in mind. Following adequate treatment with penicillin, survival from infection will result in most, but for those sustaining rupture of the aortic valve, the prognosis is grave, the majority succumbing with left ventricular failure within six months.

Only since the advent of penicillin has recovery from pneumococcal endocarditis been possible and the minimal amount of this antibiotic requisite for cure is unknown. A recovery following treatment with less than 300,000 units of penicillin a day is included in this series and in terms of present day usage, this is not a large amount of antibiotic. In patients with aortic insufficiency of uncertain origin, the possibility of healed pneumococcal endocarditis merits consideration along with other unusual causes of this lesion and a history of pneumococcal infection should be sought.

Conclusions

A review of the history of pneumococcal endocarditis points to the probable failure of normal phagocytic mechanisms in endocardial infection and to the need for a bactericidal agent to effect cure of such infection. Treatment with penicillin enables survival from pneumococcal endocarditis but may fail to prevent rupture of the aortic valve as a sequel to valvular injury from infection prior to therapy. Patients surviving infection but sustaining rupture of the aortic valve usually develop cardiac failure and have a poor prognosis. The frequent association of pneumococcal endocarditis and meningitis has been noted and the importance of examining patients with pneumococcal meningitis for evidence of endocardial lesions has been stressed.

Acknowledgments. Appreciation is expressed to Dr. A. McGehee Harvey, Physician-in-Chief, and to Dr. Arnold R. Rich, Pathologist-in-Chief, The Johns Hopkins Hospital, Baltimore, Maryland, for permission to include in this report clinical and pathological data relating to Cases #1, #2 and #3.

References

1. Heschl: Pathologisch-Anatomische Mittheilungen aus dem Gratzer allgemeinen Krankenhause. 4. Zur Casuistik und Aetiologie der Endocarditis (Fortsetzung). Oesterr. Zeitschr. f. pract. Heilkunde. 8 Jahrg. 238, 1862.

2. Osler, W.: Infectious (So-Called Ulcerative) Endocarditis. Arch. Med. 5: 44, 1881.

3. Netter: De l'Endocardite Végétante-Ulcereuse d'Origine Pneumonique. Arch. de Physiol. norm. et path. 8 (3rd series): 106, 1886.

4. Preble, H. B.: Pneumococcus Endocarditis. Am. J. Med. Sc. 128: 782, 1904.

5. Thomas, H. M., Jr. and O'Hara, D.: Pneumococcus Type I Vegetative Endocarditis. Report of a Case Following an Attack of Lobar Pneumonia. Bull. Johns Hopkins Hosp. 31: 417, 1920.

6. Wadsworth, A. B. and Sickles, G. M.: A Study of Pneumococci Isolated from Horses Undergoing Pneumococcus Immunization. J. Exp. Med. 45: 787, 1927.

7. Heffron, R.: Pneumonia with Special Reference to Pneumococcus Lobar Pneumonia, The Commonwealth Fund, New York, 1939, p. 592.

13

The Role of Toxemia and of Neural Injury in the Outcome of Pneumococcal Meningitis

The availability of antimicrobial drugs has affected not only the morbidity and mortality of infectious diseases but also the opportunities for the physician to increase his understanding of them. By altering profoundly the course of many infections, drugs may make it difficult or impossible for the contemporary investigator to study their natural history; for the withholding of therapy from man could scarcely be justified. Contrariwise, in certain other infections, marked by fatality rates approaching 100 percent in the absence of therapy, the prolongation of life or recovery which follows the administration of effective remedies may permit further insight into those factors which affect prognosis. In the case of pneumococcal disease, several examples may be cited. The biological differences in the evolution of pneumonia and bacteremia caused by different pneumococcal types have been highlighted strikingly by therapy with penicillin,[1] and the varying efficacy of phagocytic mechanisms in different anatomical sites has been brought out by the use of bacteriostatic and bactericidal drugs in the treatment of pneumonia and of endocarditis[2] caused by the same organism. The administration of penicillin in the treatment of pneumococcal meningitis has modified significantly the course of this infection also and the results thereof have suggested several factors which may play a role in the evolution of this disorder.

Prior to the advent of the sulfonamides, pneumococcal meningitis was an almost uniformly fatal disorder, and the occasional recoveries which did occur were considered in many instances sufficiently unusual to prompt their reporting in medical periodicals. The role of bacteremia as a determinant of the outcome of infection, however, received little attention; for most patients succumbed whether it were present or absent. Following the introduction of the sulfonamides, the prognosis of the patient with pneumococcal meningitis was moderately but definitely improved. At this time, divergent views concerning the effect of bacteremia on the outlook for recovery began to be expressed,[3,4] and these differences of view were not resolved entirely even during the early years in which penicillin was available. In collating the data from many reports, however, Ruegsegger[5] came to the conclusion that bacteremia was a factor affecting prognosis and also that patients with meningitis following pneumococcal infection of the upper respiratory tract and its appendages had a better chance of recovery than those whose meningeal infection was a sequel to pneumonia. Shortly thereafter, Dowling and his associates[6] described the beneficial effects of significantly larger doses of penicillin than had been administered earlier by others and established the basis for the contemporary treatment of this disorder. The observations to be reported are based upon a group of 64 patients with pneumococcal meningitis, all of whom received 12 million units of penicillin or more a day by continuous intravenous infusion, save three bacteremic patients who died within five hours of hospitalization.

It has been usual, in the past, in analyzing the effect of bacteremia upon prognosis, to consider all cases of pneumococcal meningitis, regardless of pathogenesis, as a single group. Differing from meningococcal meningitis, which is thought now almost always to be the sequel to colonization of the upper respiratory tract and to bacteremia,[7] pneumococcal meningitis may arise in a diversity of ways. In some patients, it appears as a complication of pneumococcal pneumonia and bacteremia. In others, it may develop following infection of the upper respiratory tract by direct extension from a paranasal sinus or from the middle ear. In this latter circumstance, bacteremia may be absent or present. It is possible, therefore, to delineate four potential groups of patients with pneumococcal meningitis: those with a cephalic portal of entry with or without bacteremia and those with a pulmonary portal of entry with or without bacteremia. It is obvious that any case of pneumococcal meningitis complicating or following pneumonia must be secondary to invasion of the circulation. Unlike meningococcal meningitis, which appears often to follow the transient occurrence of meningococcemia, pneumococcal meningitis secondary to pulmonary infection associated with negative blood cultures is a rarity in the absence of treatment and will not be considered here. In cases of pneumococcal meningitis secondary to sinusitis or to otitis, it is probable that bacteremia follows invasion of the meninges, for it appears seldom to be present in association with sinusitis or otitis alone. A search for adequately controlled clinical data relevant to this question, however, was unsuccessful.

Table 1 records the outcome of illness in 64 patients with pneumococcal meningitis classified according to the three categories just described, 61 of whom were treated with 12 million units of penicillin or more per day. The difference in outcome between the first group, with meningitis secondary to extension from a cephalic focus unaccompanied by bacteremia, and the remaining two groups, in which meningitis was associated with bacteria in the

Table 1. *The Effect of Bacteremia on Fatality in Pneumococcal Meningitis of Diverse Origins*

Clinical Findings	No. of Cases	Fatal Cases	Fatal Cases, %
Otitis or sinusitis, meningitis	13	0	0
Otitis or sinusitis, meningitis, bacteremia	27	17	63
Pneumonia, bacteremia	24	20	83

circulation, is striking. Although the groups are small, the differences between the first and second and between the first and third groups are highly significant when assessed by the small chi square test,[8] the P values being less than 0.001 in each instance. Judged by other criteria held to be of prognostic import in pneumococcal meningitis[7,9]: age (Table 2), state of consciousness (Table 3), leukocyte count and duration of illness prior to hospitalization, the patients with a primary cephalic focus and without bacteremia appear to have been somewhat less seriously ill than those in the two other groups under consideration. None of the other prognostic indices, however, serves quite so strikingly as a guide to the likelihood of recovery or death. It is of interest that the six patients with meningitis following pneumonia who had endocarditis fared no worse than the remainder of their group. It is altogether probable that, were the numbers of patients in each category larger, some deaths would be observed among those with non-bacteremic meningitis of cephalic origin; but it is unlikely that such a happenstance would negate the conclusion drawn from the available data.

In the light of the foregoing observations, the following inferences seem reasonable. It appears that, with adequate doses of a pneumococcidal drug such as penicillin, the meningeal and neural involvement can be controlled adequately in many instances. The toxemia that accompanies bacteremia at the time treatment is begun, however, is uninfluenced directly by antimicrobial therapy and plays a significant role in causing the death of bacteremic patients. That the mortality of bacteremic pneumococcal meningitis of cephalic origin is higher than that of bacteremic pneumococcal pneumonia is not surprising when one considers that the nervous system is a midline structure and, unlike the lungs, is involved usually in its entirety.

It seems, therefore, that bacteremia is of different import in pneumococcal and in meningococcal meningitis. In the latter disease, the view expressed by Dowling and his associates[7,10] that the presence or absence of bacteremia at the time of hospitalization has little, if any, effect on outcome is now held widely. It is consistent with the concept that most, if not all, cases of men-

Table 2. *Age Distribution of Patients with Pneumococcal Meningitis of Diverse Origins*

	Age			
Clinical Findings	*12–29*	*30–49*	*50+*	*50+, %*
Otitis or sinusitis, meningitis	0/4*	0/3	0/6	46
Otitis or sinusitis, meningitis, bacteremia	0/1	3/9	14/17	63
Pneumonia, bacteremia	—	5/7	15/17	71

*Numerator designates fatal cases, denominator total cases in each category.

Table 3. *State of Consciousness on Admission of Patients with Pneumococcal Meningitis of Diverse Origins*

	State of Consciousness				
Clinical Findings	*Alert*	*Con-fused*	*Stuporous*	*Un-known*	*Stu-porous, %*
Otitis or sinusitis, meningitis	0/1*	0/6	0/5	0/1	40
Otitis or sinusitis, meningitis, bacteremia	1/3	1/6	15/18	—	67
Pneumonia, bacteremia	1/1	5/7	14/15	0/1	60

*Numerator designates fatal cases, denominator total cases in each category.

ingococcal meningitis are secondary to meningococcemia. Pneumococcal meningitis, on the other hand, may be secondary either to bacteremia or to direct extension of infection from a cephalic focus. It is because of this diversity of pathogenesis that bacteremia is of different and greater significance in pneumococcal meningitis than it is in meningococcal meningitis.

One other factor of potential interest has emerged from the analysis of this group of patients. Table 4 contrasts the incidence of bacteremia complicating pneumococcal meningitis of cephalic origin with that complicating pneumococcal pneumonia in a group of patients seen contemporaneously in the same hospital. Again, the number of cases of meningitis is small, but the difference between the bacteremia rate of 28 per cent in pneumonia and that of 68 per cent in meningitis is statistically significant, P being less than 0.001.

Although controlled data in experimental animals are not available, several studies of experimental pneumococcal meningitis and of experimental pneumococcal pneumonia are consistent with the view that the barrier interposed between the subarachnoid space and the venous circulation is distinctly less

Table 4. *Incidence of Bacteremia Complicating Pneumococcal Pneumonia and Pneumococcal Meningitis of Cephalic Origin*

Illness	Total Cases	Bacteremic Cases	Bacteremic Cases, %
Pneumonia*	1074	303	28
Meningitis	40	27	68

*Types I, III, IV, VII, VIII and XII.

efficient than that which tends to block the passage of bacteria from the pulmonary lymphatics into the thoracic duct and subclavian vein. In experimental lobar pneumonia in the dog, Robertson and his colleagues[11-13] reported an incidence of bacteremia of 52 percent following the intrabronchial instillation of large inocula of pneumococcus Type I or II, a value considerably higher than that observed in naturally acquired infection, which is probably initiated with fewer organisms, in man. Petersdorf and Luttrell,[14] producing experimental meningitis in the same animal with pneumococcus Type III by inoculation of the subarachnoid space, found an incidence of bacteremia of 72 percent in a group of 75 dogs infected successfully. Of equal interest is the fact that, among 15 animals inoculated by the same technique which failed to develop meningitis, none had bacteremia. This latter observation suggests strongly that bacteremia in these animals was the sequel to infection of the subarachnoid space rather than the result of contamination of the circulation arising from the method of inoculation.

Investigations of the relationship of the cerebrospinal fluid to the blood vascular circulation during the past decade fit well with the clinical and experimental observations cited. Studies of the absorption of red blood cells labeled with radioactive isotopes (P^{32} and Cr^{51}) from the subarachnoid space have shown the absence of radioactivity from the cervical lymph nodes and the appearance in the circulation of tagged cells whether or not the cervical lymphatics were ligated.[15, 16] That some material introduced into the subarachnoid space may find its way into lymphatic channels may be demonstrated with dye-labeled protein,[17] but this pathway of egress from the confines of the central nervous system appears not to be the principal one. Of considerable interest are the more recent anatomical and physiological studies of the arachnoid villi by Welch and his associates.[18, 19] Perfusion of the excised dura and saggital sinus of monkeys at physiological pressures showed that fluid passed only in one direction, from the subarachnoid space into the saggital sinus. At comparable pressures, yeast cells and erythrocytes could be demonstrated to pass, in the same direction, from one side of the membrane to the other. Anatomical studies of the expanded arachnoid villi showed them to be composed of a complex of tube-like structures in a valved arrangement accounting for the findings observed in the perfusion experiments. It appears, therefore, that a pathway exists for the ready passage of bacteria from the subarachnoid space into the circulation when elevation of cerebrospinal fluid pressure exists. In the light of these circumstances, it might be anticipated that patients with pneumococcal meningitis of cephalic origin and bacteremia would have higher cerebrospinal fluid pressures than those with the same disorder unaccompanied by bacteremia. Because of the many factors which influence the clinical measurement of cerebrospinal fluid pressure, it is doubtful that much reliance can be placed on the data obtained from a retrospective study, and it would be desirable to collect additional information with the preceding hypothesis in mind. It is of some interest, however, that the average cerebrospinal fluid pressure of the patients with meningitis of cephalic origin and bacteremia was 100 mm higher than that of their counterparts lacking bacteremia.

In conclusion, the observation of a small group of patients with pneumococcal meningitis of diverse pathogenesis suggests that the presence or absence of bacteremia and of the toxemia associated with it have a significant influence on prognosis in this disease. It appears also that the anatomical barriers to the spread of infection from the meninges to the blood vascular circulation are significantly less efficient than those interposed between the lung and the blood stream. Analysis of additional cases of pneumococcal meningitis in the manner described will be helpful in supporting or modifying these views.

References

1. Austrian, R. The Current Status of Bacteremic Pneumococcal Pneumonia. Reevaluation of an Under-emphasized Clinical Problem. *Trans. Assoc. Am. Phys. 76*: 117–124, 1963.

2. Austrian, R. Pneumococcal Endocarditis, Meningitis, and Rupture of the Aortic Valve. *A.M.A. Arch. Int. Med. 99*: 539–544, 1957.

3. Keefer, C. S. The Treatment of Bacterial Meningitis. *Med. Cl. N. Amer. 25*: 1287–1315, 1941.

4. Waring, G. W. and Weinstein, L. The Treatment of Pneumococcal Meningitis. *Am. J. Med. 5*: 402–418, 1948.

5. Ruegsegger, J. M. Pneumococcal Meningitis. A Review. *U.S. Naval Med. Bull. 49*: 1159–1168, 1949.

6. Dowling, H. F., Sweet, L. K., Robinson, J. A., Zellers, W. W. and Hirsh, H. L.

The Treatment of Pneumococcic Meningitis with Massive Doses of Systemic Penicillin. *Am. J. Med. Sc. 217*: 149–156, 1949.

7. Dowling, H. F. The Acute Bacterial Diseases, Their Diagnosis and Treatment. W. B. Saunders Co., Phila. and London, 1948, pp. 202–226.

8. Hill, A. B. Principles of Medical Statistics. The Lancet Ltd., London, 1937, pp. 92–93.

9. Carpenter, R. R. and Petersdorf, R. G. The Clinical Spectrum of Bacterial Meningitis. *Am. J. Med. 33*: 262–275, 1962.

10. Lepper, M. H., Sweet, L. K. and Dowling, H. F. Treatment of Meningococcic Infections with Sulfadiazine and Sulfamerazine (Sulfamethyldiazine, Monomethylsulfadiazine). *J.A.M.A. 123*: 134–138, 1943.

11. Terrell, E. E., Robertson, O. H. and Coggeshall, L. T. Experimental Pneumococcus Lobar Pneumonia in the Dog. I. Method of Production and Course of the Disease. *J. Clin. Invest. 12*: 393–432, 1933.

12. Robertson, O. H., Coggeshall, L. T. and Terrell, E. E. Experimental Pneumococcus Lobar Pneumonia in the Dog. II. Pathology. *J. Clin. Invest. 12*: 433–466, 1933.

13. Robertson, O. H., Coggeshall, L. T. and Terrell, E. E. Experimental Pneumococcus Lobar Pneumonia in the Dog. III. Pathogenesis. *J. Clin. Invest. 12*: 467–493, 1933.

14. Petersdorf, R. G. and Luttrell, C. N. Studies on the Pathogenesis of Meningitis. I. Intrathecal Infection. *J. Clin. Invest. 41*: 311–319, 1962.

15. Simmonds, W. J. The Absorption of Labelled Erythrocytes from the Subarachnoid Space in Rabbits. *Austral. J. Exp. Biol. Med. Sc. 31*: 77–83, 1953.

16. Adams, J. E. and Prawiroherdja, S. Fate of red blood cells injected into cerebrospinal fluid pathways. *Neurology 9*: 561–564, 1959.

17. Courtice, F. C. and Simmonds, W. J. The Removal of Protein from the Subarachnoid Space. *Austral. J. Exp. Biol. Med. Sc. 29*: 255–263, 1951.

18. Welch, K. and Friedman, V. The Cerebrospinal Fluid Valves. *Brain 83*: 454–469, 1960.

19. Welch, K. and Pollay, M. Perfusion of particles through arachnoid villi of the monkey. *Am. J. Physiol. 201*: 651–654, 1961.